The Lyme Disease Survival Guide

The Lyme Disease Survival Guide

Physical, Lifestyle and Emotional Strategies for Healing

With a Dash of Humor to Light the Way

By Connie Strasheim

Foreword by James Schaller, M.D.

BioMed Publishing Group

BioMed Publishing Group
P.O. Box 9012
South Lake Tahoe, CA 96158
www.LymeBook.com

Copyright 2008 by Connie Strasheim
ISBN 10: 0-9763797-4-0
ISBN 13: 978-0-9763797-4-4
Cover design by Connie Strasheim.
Cover painting by Julie Strasheim.
Author photographs by Steve Sokolik.

For related books and DVDs visit us online at www.LymeBook.com.

Disclaimer

The author is not a physician or doctor, and this book is not intended as medical advice. It is also not intended to prevent, diagnose, treat or cure disease. Instead, the book is intended only to share the author's research, as would an investigative journalist. The book is provided for informational and educational purposes only, not as treatment instructions for any disease.

Lyme Disease is a dangerous disease and requires treatment by a licensed physician; this book is not a substitute for professional medical care. The statements in this book have not been evaluated by the FDA.

Acknowledgements

To my friend Rick R., for encouraging me in God's love, and for never leaving nor forsaking me, no matter how many tears I cried. To Mom and Dad, for bearing the constant burden of my pain and hardship over the past few years. For providing for me financially when I was penniless, and lending an ear in moments of grief. To Wendy and Julie, my beloved sisters, for your compassion and understanding. To my friend Kristin Z., for your wisdom and friendship. To Phil, Avril, Jnanda, Jamie, Troy, Brad, Meredith, Dana and all of my friends who have suffered alongside me with Lyme disease; your companionship has been like a warm blanket for my soul. To Mark, April, Julie, Jason, Kathleen, Steve and all of my friends from the Upside Down Kingdom Bible study; thank you for listening to me every Thursday night during the most difficult year of my life. To David R., for encouraging me to start a blog. To my Aunts Sandy, Simone and Kathey, and my friend Susan H., for your love, encouragement and helping me with my jewelry business when I was too sick to work.

To Dr. A. LaBair, for being the one to diagnose me with Lyme disease. I might have continued wandering in the wilderness for years if it hadn't been for you. To G. Blier, Dr. R. Loyd, Dr. E. Hesse-Sheehan, Dr. C. Fletcher, and M. Fett; thank you for your compassion and amazing work which have brought me ever closer to the door of health. To Dr. Schaller, Dr. LaBair and Dr. Hesse-Sheehan; thank you for your support during the project.

To Bryan Rosner, my publisher, thank you for helping me to share my voice with the world.

To all of the healthcare practitioners who are dedicated to treating those with Lyme disease: Thank you for healing and helping where others have not. May those who are ignorant about what they suffer one day find hope through people like you.

And to Jesus Christ, my best friend, my Savior and my hope—I could not have made it through this battle without You. May You forever be praised for your tireless love towards me and humanity.

Table of Contents

Foreword by James Schaller, M.D. 1

What is this Book About? 3

My Healing Testimony 4

What You Know About this Illness Could Be All Wrong..............................9

SECTION I:
PHYSICAL STRATEGIES FOR HEALING LYME DISEASE

Chapter 1 Protocols for Healing Lyme Disease 17

Finding Your Healing Path in a Labyrinth of Possibilities 17

Seven Primary Protocols Defined 18

MMS—Miracle Mineral Supplement, the Latest (and Greatest?) Pathogen Killer.......21

Can Your Body Heal Itself? The Power Behind Immune Response Training.............. 22

Changing Your Cellular Behavior with Quantum Techniques 23

Bioresonance and Similar Energy Therapies... 25

Formulating a Pharmaceutical Antibiotic Plan to Combat Borrelia 27

Herbal and Pharmaceutical Remedies for Babesia, Bartonella and Ehrlichia............. 29

Beat Lyme Disease with the Electromagnetic Energy of Rife Machines..................... 32

Colloidal Silver, a Tested and True Antimicrobial Remedy.................................... 34

Treating Your Mold and Candida to Heal from Lyme Disease.............................. 35

Chapter 2 Detoxification Strategies 39

The Liver.. 39
  Cleansing with Beets and Coffee *39*
  Another Easygoing Flush *40*
  Unloading the Liver's Burden with Nutrients *41*
The Skin, Kidneys and Lymphatic System... 43
  Cleansing the Kidneys with Tea and Herbs... *43*
  Sweating Out Toxins with Sauna Therapy.. *44*
  Helping Traffic on Your Lymphatic Highway with Body Brushing *45*
Additional Strategies 46
  Eliminating Stealth Toxins from Your Diet and Household................................ *46*
  The Deleterious Effects of Neurotoxins and How to Remove Them..................... *48*
  Factors Affecting Your Body's Ability to Remove Toxins *49*

Chapter 3 Testing for Infections 53

How to Determine Whether You Have Lyme Disease and its Co-Infections.............. 53

The Newest Testing Methods: Flow Cytometry and Immunoflourescent Assay 57

How Do You Know if a Supplement Is Right for You? Learning to Muscle Test..........58

Chapter 4 Hormone Balance 63

The Healing Power and Dangerous Potential of Supplemental Cortisol 63

The Fussy Thyroid and How to Fix It 65

Causes of, and Solutions for, Hypothalamic-Pituitary-Adrenal Foul-Ups 66

Optimizing Insulin, Adrenaline and Cortisol Function and Production 68

The Link Between Adrenal Fatigue and Hypothyroidism and Why It Matters...........70

Chapter 5 Adjunct Lyme Disease Treatments............. 73

Nutrients for Immune Function 73

Fixing a Broken Lyme Heart with Herbal Remedies and Other Nutrients...........73

Cordyceps Mushrooms for Energy, Immune Support, and More 74

Treating Multiple Symptoms with Japanese Knotweed 75

Enzymes and other Solutions for Thick Blood 76

Super Siberian Ginseng for Mood, Stamina and Immune Function 77

Natural Anti-Inflammatory Treatments 78

*Enhancing Immune Cell Production with Transfer Factor, Glutathione & More.*79

Boosting the Body with Stem Cell Enhancers 81

Increasing Iron Stores to Combat Babesia 82

Supplemental Oxygen for Life and Lyme.. 83

Other Adjunct Healing Strategies.. 84

Dying for Some zzz's: Causes of, and Solutions for, Insomnia 84

Fantastic Fixes for Low Energy...87

Decreasing Your Symptoms by Increasing Serotonin.. 89

Zoning in on the Ozone... 90

Avoiding Damaging Electromagnetic Fields 91

The Benefits of Sunshine 92

The Perils of Tap Water and Finding A Suitable Water Filtration System 93

Chapter 6 Protocol Considerations 95

Distinguishing Herxes from Flare-ups and Relapses..95

To Combine or Not to Combine Protocols, That Is the Question 98

Should You Pulse and Rotate Herbs, or Take Long-Term? 100

Getting the Most out of Herbal and Vitamin Supplements..102

Why It's Good to Blast Critters on the Full Moon 103

You Don't Need to Know about Every Little Infection in Your Body to Heal.............104

Trusting Your Gut when Making a Game Plan...106

Getting Rid of the Inner Quack and Learning to Trust Alternative Medicine 107

Chapter 7 Heavy Metals...................................... 111

The Importance of Ridding the Body of Heavy Metals 111

The Power of Minerals to Remove Metals 113

SECTION 2:
LIFESTYLE STRATEGIES FOR HEALING LYME DISEASE

Chapter 8 Diet and Supplements 117

Self-discipline in Your Diet 117
Avoiding Harmful Food Additives by Learning the Language of Deception 119
So Many Lyme Diets, So Much Confusion: Choosing a Regimen that Works 120
Becoming Liberated from Pill Fatigue 122
The Benefits of Maté 124

Chapter 9 Exercise 127

An Exercise Plan that Will Get You Moving but Won't Leave You Wiped Out 127

Chapter 10 Relationships 129

"I'm too Sick to Be in a Romantic Relationship" ... Or Are You, Really? 129
They Will Never Understand: Accepting Your Family's And Friends' Limitations 133
Lessons of Dating from a Disastrous Night Out 136

Chapter 11 Finances and Work 143

No Dough to Throw at Lyme Disease: Formulating a Protocol on a Budget 143
To Get a Job or Not Get a Job 145

Chapter 12 Travel 149

Tips for Airplane Travel when You're Symptomatic 149

Chapter 13 Helping Others 157

We All Advocate what Works for Us: Take Care when Leading Another To Health .. 157
Energy and Spoons: Chronic Fatigue Sufferers Don't Get Much Silverware 158

Chapter 14 Habits 161

Keeping a Lyme Log to Track Your Progress 161
The Problem with, and Usefulness of, "To-Do" Lists 163
The Dangers of Leading a High Cortisol Lifestyle 164

Chapter 15 For the Day-to-Day 167

Must Your Life Be All About Lyme Disease? Ways to Get Out of Your Head............. 167

Energy versus Hyperactivity and Learning to Slow Down... 169

The Necessity of a Multi-faceted Approach to Healing... 171

The Power of Environment to Heal 172

Taking a Vacation from Illness to Enjoy Life.. 174

Forty Little Lessons of Lyme Disease 175

Chapter 16 And for a Little Humor... 179

Ten Reasons Why You Should Be a Professional Sofa Spud.. 179

The Lyme Disease Store: Finding a Few Goofy Things to Take Home with You........ 181

Twenty Things to Do on a Date When You Both Have Lyme Disease 185

How a Lymie Makes a Salad: Blunders of a Lyme Body in Action............................ 187

Morning Malaise and the Bed Battle with the Body...189

Seven Advantages to Living in Costa Rica with Lyme Disease 193

SECTION III:
EMOTIONAL STRATEGIES FOR HEALING LYME DISEASE

Chapter 17 Managing Circumstantial Difficulties 197

Eat Your Peas! I mean, "P's"...Those that Stand for Perseverance and Patience 197

Remembering that Your Brain Still Works on "Stupid" Days.................................... 199

Pay Attention to the Small Changes When You're Fed Up with Your Regimen 200

Grieving Over a Life Lost and the Humdrum of Existence 201

"Will I EVER Get Better?"...Hope for When You Crash... 203

Focusing on Nine Lessons of Chronic Illness.. 204

The Fun House Monster...Hope for When You're on a Wild Mental Ride 206

Chapter 18 The Power of Belief, Thought & Words.. 209

Get Healthy by Getting out of Victim Mode 209

Telling Your Truth to the World...Your Health May Depend Upon It...................... 212

Vanquishing Fear: the Sneaky, Slow Killer...213

Is Your Subconscious Keeping You Sick?...The Truth Behind Blocks to Healing 216

How Words Alter Your Physical Reality 217

Creating an Alphabet Soup of Abundance in Your Life...218

Countering Despairing Thoughts with Affirmations...219

"But I Deserve to Be Well!"...How a Spirit of Entitlement Fosters Misery.................222

"Why Me?"...Don't Even Ask the Question 223

Sub-personalities of the Anxious Lyme Disease Sufferer 224

Visualizations for Healing...Two Mind-Body Techniques 228

Chapter 19 Strategies that Go Beyond the Mind....... 233

Releasing Emotional Trauma from the Body with Neuro-Emotional Technique...... 233

Reprogramming the Subconscious Mind to Rewire Your Cellular Behavior 235

Chapter 20 The Moral of the Story...........................237

Lessons from the Food Stamp Office...Don't Buy into Lies about Who You Are 237

For One Hour, I Didn't Have Lyme...Forgetting Your Limitations & Forging Ahead 242

Sauna Talk, Part One...Learning to Share Lyme Disease with the World 243

Sauna Talk Part II...Learning to Keep Life in Perspective 247

Appendix: Spiritual Lessons Based on My Personal Belief in a God Who Heals 253

    Born to Fly, but Stuck in Jail...Finding Freedom in a Life that Feels Confining 253

    The Redemptive Potential of Illness and the Power of God to Make it Happen . 255

    Finding Peace and Joy through Pain and Suffering 259

    Learning to Long for God, First and Foremost 260

    Why Won't God Heal Me? 264

Bibliography 267

Lyme-Related Product Catalog from BioMed Publishing Group 271

Foreword by James Schaller, M.D.

Connie is a real writer so you will not struggle to read this book. She is a careful intellectual health explorer, so like a top quality Sci-Fi thriller, get ready to go to new and cutting-edge places to increase your health. If you are looking for depressing complaints—find another book. Connie offers increasing humor with every section and yet she "gets it". She knows that most health care practitioners do not "get it", and she has had to deal with medical nonsense just like you. She is not afraid of reality, but offers you hope. And when you are done, you will feel like she is a close friend. She has the remarkable ability to bring power and strength to your spine if you feel disheartened.

Connie covers it all and offers many types of options to fit every health care taste. If you expect to agree with her on every page, please appreciate that if you looked in the mirror, you would not even agree with your own beliefs from last year. Indeed, since publishing both of my books on Babesia and Artemisia last year, I have found that my dosing of Mepron and Artesunate is too low to cure Babesia. So I do not even agree with the beliefs that I held a mere twelve months ago. But you will receive many options and new ideas from Connie which are being talked about and used presently in many progressive health circles.

You will get the most from her book if you let her light and warm personality roll over you as you read, and in terms of content, simply explore those areas which you feel are advances that YOU want to pursue. Connie is so broad she can offer 20 "specials" at the same time, like they do in fine restaurants. I cannot imagine that anyone in the USA could not learn some important things from this book. Much of it is very new and only out in recent months.

She understands that co-infections matter, and without treatment of the more important ones, like Bartonella or Babesia, complete recovery from Lyme is probably impossible. She does not confuse lowering body volume of an infection with curing illness. She understands that most tests for the thirty-two species of Bartonella are useless.

Connie understands healing can come in many forms, such as traditional antibiotics, enhancement of immunity, removing body-stress pollution, anti-inflammatory food, faith to lift you from beneath a bad health week, and herbs. Indeed, I have found in

Connie Strasheim

intimate partnership with my treasured "brother" Ching Zhang M.D., that new doses of Artemisia—in the form of artesunate and the HH Chinese combination herbs, are curative for Babesia and Bartonella—just not at previously lower doses. The world has already decided that Artemisia derivatives are the cure for malaria, which affects 400 million/year. Connie gets this reality. She knows that many new interventions to cure tick and flea -borne infections will require new sources of powerful and effective treatments. We have proven just this in our blinded research on some herbs. This research is currently in the process of being published in stages.

If you are looking for simplistic guidelines or "protocols" Connie will not offer them. She is too smart to believe in clone medicine. She knows 7-minute routine medical sessions do not bring cure or any sense of humanity to a reader. And that is the point, in coming to know this precious wise explorer, you will feel more alive and hopeful, as you get to know her and read her fine work. Sure, you will learn some new ideas and new medicine and treatment options. But her book's aftertaste is hope and contentment. And that alone is well worth the price of "admission."

In writing this book, she has secluded herself like the great writers of past generations have. In a remote region of Costa Rica, a place of passionate dedicated study, Connie has utterly immersed herself in the world of healing tick-borne infections. I am pleased to finally see this caterpillar emerge as a butterfly of hope, with useful options to offer the world.

Now come to the buffet and see what parts you want to enjoy.

James Schaller, MD, MAR
www.personalconsult.com

Author of 27 Journal Publications and 25 Books
Published or Pending Books Include:

The Diagnosis and Treatment of Babesia
The 16 Reasons Lyme Disease Treatment Fails
30 Unique Bartonella Skin Findings to Aid in Diagnosis
Mold Illness and Mold Remediation Made Simple
ADD, ODD and Youth Behavior Problems: 100 Solutions Sincere Doctors Miss
When Traditional Medicine Fails
The Diagnosis and Treatment of Bartonella
The Definitive Guide to Artemisia Derivatives for Babesia, Malaria and Cancer
Suboxone: Take Your Life Back From Pain Medicines

What Is this Book About?

Offering a holistic approach to healing, this book provides not only information on treatments for the physical body, but also strategies for healing the mind and spirit, at the same time that it entertains and supplies practical lifestyle suggestions for coping with illness. Divided into sections, the first part describes physical strategies, with information on the most widely used protocols to treat Lyme disease in conventional and (especially) alternative medicine. Information on detoxification and supportive strategies is included and, while not comprehensive, is intended to provide an overview of different treatments that have historically been beneficial for healing others from Lyme disease. The second and third parts of the book, borne out of my own struggles with the illness, are intended to offer insights into the lifestyle and emotional challenges of illness as well as solutions for these. Two final sections on humor and spirituality are to lift your spirits and suggest the role of God in healing. While written from a Christian perspective, people of other faiths may yet appreciate the last section, which ponders, among other things, the redemptive potential of illness and God's great love for humanity.

While informative, this book also entertains, and is sprinkled with humor and occasional irony. I know of no other way to write about such a sober topic as Lyme disease. The lifestyle and emotional sections, in particular, are laced with dry wit because it's a powerful way for me to be able to say to others, "I know what you're feeling because I've been there, too."

While no two people will have the same healing path, I share my personal experience and research with the hope that I can impart a tidbit of light to those who may find humor and healing in some of the strategies I present henceforth. While I have attempted to include the most recent, updated information on physical strategies, in the world of Lyme disease things quickly change, and new treatments are constantly being developed. Bear this in mind as you read. May God bless you and keep you, and may He make His face to shine upon you as you journey towards health.

Connie Strasheim

My Healing Testimony

With a shattering greeting, illness broke down the door of my life on September 26, 2004. I still recall the contents of my suitcase as I packed for a trip that evening, my heart thumping off-key, my thoughts random and my body in iron chains as if I'd already worked three fourteen-hour days at my job with United Airlines. The memory of granola bars, tucked in-between uniform shirts, along with my in-flight handbook, still haunts me. These things marked the end of an exciting life filled with activity, ambition and jaunts around the planet—and the beginning of what would become the most significant trial of my existence.

For a year following that devastating night in September, I believed that my life was over. Now, as my third anniversary with illness has come and gone, and I've lost my home, job, savings and the ability to climb mountains, I realize that, indeed, illness has destroyed life as I once knew it. However, had I known then what I know now about my god's intent and ability to heal me, from the inside out, I might not have soaked my carpet with so many tears. Had I known then that my journey with Lyme disease would teach me more in three years than thirty years of simply surviving ever could, the edges of its devastation might have been dulled. Had I realized that being pronounced a Lyme disease sufferer was only to give a name to the plethora of infections and biochemical screw-ups in my body, I would have looked more deeply and differently at healing from the beginning, and started my journey in a different place.

Or maybe, even knowing these things, I would have been devastated anyway. Chronic illness meant the death of life as I knew it, and I had to mourn the loss of that life. During the first year, grief consumed me, as hours of Internet research left me with an abundance of questions and even more answers that I suddenly had to juggle like an inexperienced clown on the edge of a nervous breakdown.

Physicians and well-meaning acquaintances who wore white lab coats of self-righteousness fueled my grief and rage. Thankfully, some of my friends and family tried to understand how the myriad of bizarre symptoms affected me. But after a couple of years, I realized that, unless another could jump into my body, nobody would ever know what this insanity was like and that I needed to stop with the expectations. Another lesson I learned early on in the journey was that no physician, shaman or PhD counselor could ever be in charge of my healing, and I'd be a fool to entrust any health care provider with that commission. They could only provide me with insights, but ultimately healing was up to my god, whose wisdom in my spirit would provide me with the information I'd need to make wise choices along the healing path.

For me, healing has required more than simply eradicating borrelia, the Lyme disease bacteria. As most chronic Lyme disease sufferers, I have at least a couple dozen other infections. Bugs are wily, opportunistic organisms. When they realize that the immune system is down, they then have a party and invite ten thousand of their best friends over. But it's okay, because I'm noticing that as my body deals with all of the other factors that have contributed to its breakdown, getting rid of the pesky infections is becoming easier.

My treatment plan has involved spending a year and a half with a Rife (Doug) machine, two years on a sea salt and vitamin C protocol, while concurrently and intermittently ingesting herbs and pharmaceutical antibiotics as I detoxified my body with saunas, enemas and agents such as chlorella and PCA-Rx. While all of these strategies, taken together, have brought me moderate improvement, after two years of treatments, my progress stagnated, and I realized that I needed to shift my focus elsewhere. Don't get me wrong. Ridding the body of pathogens is vital, as is keeping the body's detoxification pathways and other systems functioning as smoothly as possible—but it's only part of what I, and many others have needed to do in order to heal.

The other part has meant altering my lifestyle and healing emotional trauma through the use of prayer, affirmations, cranial-sacral therapy, Immune Response Training, Quantum Techniques and other mind-body strategies. It's also meant getting rid of my synthetic diet, grievous relationships, troublesome thoughts and a harried daily routine, among other environmental toxins.

Connie Strasheim

Like many Lyme disease sufferers, I would need an encyclopedia to document all of the vitamins and herbs I've taken in attempt to get this neuron or that hormone to function properly, to kill this bacteria or that virus, to detoxify this kidney or unclog that lymphatic zone. My kitchen used to look like a pharmacy, and I often wondered if I could put the local Pharma-Kia down the street out of business. My supplemental nutrient protocol has been ever changing, but has always included chlorella for detoxification, a multivitamin, fish oil, Concentrace minerals, magnesium, bio-identical thyroid hormone (T3) and melatonin for sleep.

What all the ingestants have taught me is that no one vitamin, herb or drug is a miracle-worker. What all of the other therapies have taught me is that, in conjunction with one another, they can be powerful and work best in an environment that is as free of toxins as possible, whether these be emotional, chemical or electromagnetic. What God has taught me is that healing is ultimately up to Him (Pardon my grammar, but my god likes for me to refer to him with a capital "H"). Also, that health resides not in the place of a drug or a hormone as much as in the ability to give and receive His love.

Whereas I once believed that this trial of illness was about discovering cures for chronic fatigue and Lyme disease, I now believe that it has more to do with being transformed from the inside out. God allowed my old life to die so that I could be given a new one, filled with greater purpose and peace. This life would teach me more about how to love myself and others, even though getting to that place would, paradoxically, require deep suffering.

Fortunately, over the past year and a half, life has become tolerable, even joyous at times, whereas during my first two years of total incapacitation by Lyme disease, I often felt as though I'd been given an early ticket to Hell. Since then, my body, and especially my mind, have healed exponentially, and I have begun to believe with more than a fraction of my heart that God intends to use this difficult experience for my good.

I surmise that Immune Response Training and Quantum Techniques are the most effective therapies I have undertaken thus far, because they address healing on a holistic level. Unbeknownst to me before my experience with Lyme disease, I now know that emotional trauma can be stored in organs and tissues besides the brain, and I have found it vital to treat this aspect of illness in order to eradicate the infections in my body.

S.H. Buhner's and Dr. D. Klinghardt's herbal protocol have been useful for lowering my pathogen load, and I experienced strong Jarisch-Herxheimer, or die-off reactions, from herbs such as andrographis and ozonated rizol oils containing artemisia, thyme, oregano and garlic.

The salt/C protocol, which requires taking high doses of sea salt and vitamin C to dehydrate borrelia organisms and boost the immune system, has been another helpful adjunct and was one of the first strategies I used to treat Lyme disease. It rid me of tachycardia and possibly helped with other problems. The cardiac die-off symptoms I experienced on the salt/C protocol lasted for six months. After that, I never experienced a skipped heartbeat again.

Finally, Rifing with a Doug machine produced minimal changes in my symptom picture, although I often experienced depression after sessions with the machine, which indicates that it produced herxheimer reactions and was therefore useful to an undefined extent.

I used pharmaceutical antibiotics for only a few months, in part because they severely weakened my body, and I developed a candida infection, which is not uncommon in those who decide upon this type of treatment.

My healing journey has required all the resources of my mind, body and soul. Attempting to attain wellness has been a full-time job, requiring a tenacious refusal to give up, no matter how stiff the discipline required to follow a regimen, and no matter how many times I've suffered mini-relapses despite months and months of stringent adherence to treatment protocols.

Connie Strasheim

Healing has also meant discovering and ridding myself of subconscious beliefs that have kept me rooted in illness, such as the lie that my symptoms somehow protect me from the evils of the world or that I can better get my needs met through illness. The subconscious mind operates powerfully in the mechanisms of illness, and I have had to delve deep into my soul and ask myself many questions, including whether I believe that I am truly worthy of health. I believe that much of chronic illness stems from mistaken or harmful beliefs we hold towards ourselves and other people. Prayer and bio-energetic therapies, to name a couple of methods, have helped me to discern what below-the-surface motivations have been factors in my illness.

While changing my thought patterns and lifestyle has been a tedious and often overwhelming process, the benefits I'm starting to reap from my efforts have made the journey worth it, even though I have failed in my discipline, slipped and broken my will a multitude of times. I haven't yet reached the top of the Health Mountain, but I'm on an upward slope, climbing ever higher, and at peace, knowing that with each day, I am one step closer to victory.

Paradigm-Shifting Facts about Lyme Disease: What You Know about this Illness Could Be All Wrong

If you aren't a well-read Lyme disease warrior, you might as well toss all those rumors you've heard about this illness to the bugs.

Lyme disease isn't a wee problem confined to a few states in the northeastern United States. It is everywhere, from California to Colorado to Minnesota, to Africa, Australia, Asia, Europe and Latin America. It is an epidemic in the United States and thought to be not only the fastest growing infectious disease in this country, but also the most insidious, complicated and least understood. Over three hundred species of borrelia, the bacteria that transmits Lyme disease, are known to exist worldwide, but there are probably more. Ladies and Lyme Gents, this disease is a BIG deal.

Also, Lyme disease isn't just caused by deer ticks in the northeastern United States. Fleas, mosquitoes, mites and other creepy-crawlies also carry the infection, which are harbored by a number of furry or feathered mammals, including white-footed mice, chipmunks, horses, birds and others. Not to mention your family dog, and, in fact, some Lyme disease experts believe that all dogs in the United States carry the infection. Dogs play in the grass, ticks live in the grass, and Lyme disease is everywhere. Birds are important vectors for the bacteria, spreading the illness far and wide as they cross states, countries and continents, as are people, who transmit the illness via breast milk, blood, urine, semen and other bodily fluids.

It is estimated that only one in ten Lyme disease cases is reported to the Centers for Disease Control. Further, testing and diagnosing methods are inadequate and the infection masquerades as a multitude of illnesses such as fibromyalgia, multiple sclerosis, Parkinson's and more. Thousands of cases are improperly diagnosed each year. Hence, statistics from the CDC regarding Lyme disease are grossly inaccurate, physicians are ignorant about how to diagnose and treat it, and therefore, nobody believes that it's really a problem!

Connie Strasheim

Some LLMD's (Lyme-literate medical doctors), those who have extensively researched and treated thousands of patients with Lyme disease, believe that up to twenty-five percent of the population is now infected with some species of borrelia, the bacteria which causes Lyme disease. The figure could be even higher. However, not all of these borrelia carriers will develop an active infection, as this is contingent upon other factors, including immune system function and environmental toxins.

"But I don't remember getting a tick bite." If only I had a dollar for every time I heard that one! Guess what? Most people don't remember getting bit by a tick, and most don't recall the bull's-eye rash that the bite produces. Besides, maybe you or your neighbor got Lyme from a mosquito bite.

On to the next mistaken assumption: Lyme disease doesn't (just) give you joint and cardiac problems. It can cause pain and fatigue, and it can also disable you. It affects every single organ and system of the body, and symptoms encompass and mimic those found in a multitude of illnesses. Common are headaches, brain fog and depression, dizziness, insomnia, gut pain and stiffness or paralysis of the limbs. The all-inclusive list, however, encompasses more than one hundred symptoms, and the most important of these can be found in Dr. J. Burrascano, LLMD's notes at: www.ilads.org/burrascano_1102.htm. Another site listing symptoms of Lyme disease, as well as those typical of three common Lyme disease co-infections (babesia, bartonella and ehrlichia) can be found at: www.bcclocks.com/lymebabs.html.

A review of these symptoms can help you to determine whether you have Lyme disease, though confirmation through a variety of testing methods is needed to support any clinical diagnoses since most of the symptoms can also be found in other illnesses. Conversely, chronic fatigue syndrome, fibromyalgia, multiple sclerosis, autism, Parkinson's, Alzheimer's, lupus, multiple chemical sensitivities, irritable bowel syndrome and a host of other so-called diseases may all be the "costume" that Lyme wears. Or, Lyme disease may be a factor in the instigation of other disease processes or part of the overall symptom picture that these produce.

Now, suppose you happen to detect a tick bite or notice the classic Bull's eye rash soon after being bitten by a tick. You will have to undergo six to eight weeks of antibiotic treatment. If you think two weeks or a month is sufficient, because that's what doctors typically prescribe to everyone, you should know that there has never been a study demonstrating that even thirty days of antibiotics cures the early stages of Lyme disease. However, much documentation exists to prove that short courses of antibiotics fail to eradicate the infection, even in those who immediately discover that they have been bitten by a tick and receive prompt treatment.

If you catch Lyme disease in the early stages, consider yourself lucky, because chances are excellent that you will fully recover. Some symptoms (and this is not an all-inclusive list) to watch for in the early stages include: fever, chills, stiff neck, headache, joint pain and fatigue.

If you suffer symptoms and in hindsight realize that these started shortly after you went camping in the woods a couple of months ago, and you test positive for a borrelia infection, then you are have arrived at stage two of the illness, called "early disseminated" Lyme disease. Additional symptoms to look for at this stage, in addition to those listed above, include: multiple rashes, weakness, numbness or pain in the arms or legs, an irregular heartbeat and persistent weakness or fatigue.

Weeks to months after a bug bite, arthritis (especially in the knees) and nervous system dysfunction often appear, manifesting in a myriad of symptoms and becoming more pronounced the longer a person is ill. But keep in mind that these symptom guidelines should only be loosely followed. There are no hard and fast rules, and most symptoms can manifest at any time after the tick or mosquito or bed bug has done its thing in your skin.

Connie Strasheim

To ascertain a diagnosis, forget about going to your local lab for a blood draw. Standard tests are likely to give you inaccurate results for several reasons. First, many people stop producing antibodies to Lyme disease after a period of time (especially the more chronically ill), and this is what the western blot, the most widely used lab test, measures. At least thirty percent of those with Lyme disease will test negative on it. Second, current guidelines from the powers that be don't allow for the most important bands (which refers to how the antibody appears in testing) to be recognized, which means that many positive results will be missed. IgeneX is one lab that tests for all the necessary bands, but it too has its limitations, as do all Lyme disease testing methods. And forget about the ELISA test ("ELISA" is an acronym for enzyme-linked immunosorbent assay). Like the western blot, it measures the immune system's response to an infectious agent rather than looking for foreign proteins, but for other reasons is even less accurate than the western blot.

Further, unless your doctor is a Lyme disease specialist, he or she is likely to give you a wrong interpretation of your symptoms and even your test results. Physicians just don't know enough about this disease and are not provided with the tools to make proper diagnoses. That the American Medical Association, the Centers for Disease Control and other organizations refuse to recognize the evidence that chronic Lyme disease is an epidemic and an illness that cannot be treated by a few weeks of antibiotics doesn't help doctors to make sound judgments, either.

Finally, Lyme disease isn't just about a solitary strain of bacteria. It involves multiple infections, as more often than not, borrelia doesn't travel alone and brings other microorganisms along with it into the body, each of which must be treated separately. All weaken the immune system and create multiple systemic dysfunction, thereby setting the stage for more infections to enter the body, which must also be treated.

Alternative medicine, (and it should not really be called "alternative" because doing so implies an inferior position to "traditional" medicine as we in western societies know it), offers powerful solutions for healing from Lyme disease and should be, along with traditional medicine, a foremost consideration when formulating a protocol.

It is sobering, but you must know the facts from the outset. Lyme is a difficult disease to treat; its diagnosis and treatment are complicated, but you or your loved ones *can* recover if you research, read and are dedicated to your recovery. But you must know what you are up against. The disease is a beast, and you must be willing to think outside of the box and go beyond the guidelines set by traditional medicine and its establishments in order to formulate a protocol that will heal you from the illness.

Section I

Physical Strategies for Healing Lyme Disease

Chapter 1

Protocols for Healing Lyme Disease

Finding Your Healing Path in a Labyrinth of Possibilities

Welcome to the maze! Your path will be different from that of your neighbor, who is also infected with Lyme disease, because there's no one single route to take. You might be the mouse (okay, rat) who gets put on a simple trail, but chances are, if your illness is chronic, you'll get a winding one with lots of possible detours and dead-ends. Understand this when you start out. Yes, the path of pharmaceutical antibiotics works for some. Herbs and colloidal silver may be the way for others, but don't jump on your neighbor's trail as what worked for him may not work for you.

You'll take many detours along the way, some leading you to dead ends, others bringing you closer to the exit. The only way to get to the end, however, is by scurrying along and keeping at it though your strength may fail and your heart may get discouraged.

Connie Strasheim

Eat some good cheese (rat food!) and keep your body strong however you can, for the journey is long and trying. You will pass through dark nights when you can't see the path in front of you, or won't be able to budge those back legs to get moving, but the sun will come out eventually, and, if you are willing, you'll move forward again.

Especially if you get a few other rats to encourage you and help you along.

Below are some of the more popular ways out of the labyrinth. Each one is discussed more at length later in the chapter. You are likely to find that one or more combinations of these therapies comprise your path and will be necessary in order to bring you to the exit. For some, the finish line will mean only going halfway and setting up a cozy abode inside the walled greenery of the labyrinth and being content to live with some symptoms. For them, this is their end and their freedom. For others, it will mean leaving the green walls for good.

You won't know the way out until you run the race, bump into a few walls and miss a few openings in the shrubbery, but if you keep going, you'll get there. Determination and a positive attitude are vital. You'll bump into some walls but you weren't born with a tough little skull for nothing!

Seven Primary Protocols Defined

1. **Rife machines and other devices using electromagnetic energy.** Did you know that by using an organism's electromagnetic frequency range against itself you can cause it to vibrate and shatter? This is the principle behind Rifing. By programming certain frequencies (say, 450 hertz) into a frequency generator and allowing the frequencies to pass through a contact device, you can kill Lyme spirochetes and other pathogens. Check out Bryan Rosner's book, *When Antibiotics Fail: Lyme Disease and Rife Machines, with Critical Evaluation of Leading Alternative Therapies,* for more information

on Rife machines and good adjunct therapies to try along with them (www.LymeAndRifeBook.com)

2. **Herbal antibiotics.** As powerful and effective as pharmaceutical antibiotics, (and sometimes, more so), herbs are a potent way to heal Lyme disease without damaging the body in the same way that pharmaceutical antibiotics can. Experimentation with dosages and types is necessary. Check out S.H. Buhner's book, *Healing Lyme: Natural Healing and Prevention of Lyme Borreliosis and its Coinfections;* Dr. Zhang, M.D.'s book, *Lyme Disease and Modern Chinese Medicine;* Dr. D. Klinghardt, M.D., PhD's website: www.neuraltherapy.com, or Planet Thrive: www.planetthrive.com, for more information on herbal protocols.

3. **Homeopathy.** Another powerful strategy for healing Lyme disease, and one which has taken many sufferers "out of the woods," homeopathy involves administering a small dose of a substance that, in higher doses, would cause illness in a healthy person. The idea is to stimulate the body's own healing defenses. Take a look at P. Alex and D. Smith's book, *The Homeopathic Treatment of Lyme Disease*, or R.J. Whitmond, M.D.,'s website: www.homeopathicmd.com, for more information. A good source for homeopathic remedies can be found on the Internet at: www.desertbiologicals.com.

4. **Sea Salt and Vitamin C**. This inexpensive strategy involves taking high doses of vitamin C along with sea salt and works via osmotic-induced dehydration of borrelia organisms. Salt/C is thought to be effective for all forms of borrelia, including the L-form and cystic form, and shows promise for eliminating co-infections, too. Harmless to the body, salt/C has eliminated symptoms in Lyme disease sufferers who have spent years doing antibiotics and other therapies with limited success. Take a look at these websites: www.lymephotos.com and http://www.fettnet.com/ lymestrategies/welcome.htm for more information and to find user reports from others who have employed this protocol.

Connie Strasheim

5. **Immune Response Training.** This amazing treatment involves reading codes that input healing instructions into the autonomic nervous system, which then uses the information to recognize and kill pathogens as it corrects inefficient biochemical processes. Great gains and remission from Lyme disease and other maladies have been realized with this protocol. To order a free DVD of information go to: www.lymefree.com. The founder, Gary Blier, offers a money-back guarantee if, after three sessions, you notice no change in your symptoms.

6. **Pharmaceutical Antibiotics.** This is the traditional way of treating Lyme disease in the United States. While effective for some, up to 40% of people who choose to take antibiotics relapse. This is due to, among other factors, the Lyme bacteria's developing resistance to drugs and improper administration of medication. This kind of treatment can also have long-term debilitating effects upon the immune system; however, it is indisputably the preferred method of treatment for the early stages of illness and for some, the chronic stages, as well. Check out Dr. J. Burrascano, M.D.'s notes at: www.lymediseaseassociation.org/ dbrguide200509.pdf or Dr. J. Schaller, M.D.'s website: www.hopeacademic.com for good antibiotic protocol information.

7. **Colloidal Silver.** Functions as an antibiotic and is a powerful killer of all kinds of infections, including borrelia. For more information on its use in Lyme disease, read P. Farber's, *The Micro Silver Bullet* or visit: www.silvermedicine.org.

Now, let's take a more detailed look at some of these therapies, as well as some other protocols which have proven beneficial for treating Lyme disease and its co-infections.

MMS—Miracle Mineral Supplement, the Latest (and Greatest?) Pathogen Killer

It's guinea pig time again in the Lyme disease world as bundles of sufferers try out the newest bug killer on the block, sodium chlorite (or chlorine dioxide, once it's mixed with some citric acid and hits your cells). Tested, tried and true for over 75,000 malaria victims in Africa, as well as for sufferers of other illnesses including AIDS and cancer, this amazing molecule is also showing promise for ridding sufferers of Lyme disease.

While its long-term benefits (and side effects) for healing chronic Lyme disease remain unknown, the guinea folk have so far experienced immediate, dramatic die-off reactions from its use and a reduction in symptoms. This protocol has produced symptom reductions in every single Lyme disease sufferer that I know of who has tried it. Its founder, Jim Humble, contends that MMS is the most potent pathogen killer known to man.

The key to using sodium chlorite properly is by taking it with vinegar, lemon juice, or better yet, citric acid. When this is done, chlorine dioxide is produced and utilized in a controlled, time-released fashion in the body, making it safe and effective as a pathogen killer. Although toxic when prepared commercially, when your body makes chlorine dioxide from sodium chlorite it supports the immune system, since the human body makes chlorine dioxide on its own as part of its pathogen-combating processes, anyway.

Furthermore, the chlorine dioxide ion gets used up in its action of killing pathogens, so when it has finished its work, no trace of the chemical is left behind in the body.

Rumor has it that Humble believes that it's necessary for chronic Lyme sufferers to take sodium chlorite for approximately one year in order to achieve good results, perhaps remission. I don't know if he's already tested some borrelia-infected folk for an extended period, or if this figure is his estimation based on what he knows about sodium chlorite and its actions upon pathogens. Still unknown is whether it

Connie Strasheim

can kill borrelia in cystic form, but preliminary results of its use have been encouraging.

If you decide to try out this protocol, start slowly! You never know what kind of die-off toxin fest you'll incur when this stuff hits your body. In the meantime, check in with the different on-line Yahoo! Lyme disease groups, as well as with the miracle mineral Yahoo! group, which can be found at: http://health.groups.yahoo.com/group/miracle_mineral_supplement, to learn about others' progress on the protocol. You can also report your progress to Jim by going to the MMS web site: www.miracleminéral.org, and clicking on the "contact" link. A free e-book on the protocol can also be downloaded there.

Can Your Body Heal Itself? The Power Behind Immune Response Training

Immune Response Training (IRT) is a fascinating Lyme disease remedy that bases its success upon prayer and the body's ability to heal itself.

Part of the theory behind IRT asks the question: Why give your body an outside substance when God has blessed your immune system with the ability to heal Lyme disease, along with the help of a little prayer?

According to Gary Blier, the founder of IRT, the body sometimes forgets what it's supposed to do in its day-to-day functioning. Environmental toxins and trauma cause this to happen, which is why infections are allowed to wreak havoc in the first place. When the immune system is working optimally, however, infections such as borrelia burgdorferi cannot thrive and become active.

Blier believes that the body is a remarkable organism, with the potential to eradicate any infection and to heal from any disease, if only it's reminded of what it's supposed to do. Immune Response Training can give it the nudge that it needs to get headed in the right direction.

This is done through the use of codes comprised of words, letters and numbers that make no sense to the conscious mind but which serve as instructions for the autonomic nervous system. The ANS then uses the information to alter cellular behavior. The codes are integrated into the body with the help of a CD that contains more language designed specifically for the ANS. Prayer following an IRT session seals the blessing upon the work of the codes in the body.

How do the codes work exactly? Who knows! Gary Blier would tell you that IRT is an art. While it employs concepts found in energy medicine, I believe it's a science whose principles haven't been fully conceptualized or defined by man. It's one of those things where the What or the How of a healing protocol has been given, without its inter-workings being fully revealed, even to its founder.

If you can accept the mystery behind IRT's codes and how they work, and if you believe in the power of prayer to heal, then IRT may just be right for you. We're all given a different path to walk in the journey through Lyme disease, but I can tell you from personal experience that IRT works, and it is powerful.

Changing Your Cellular Behavior with Quantum Techniques

Have you ever noticed how many folks have been brainwashed into believing that health is achieved solely through the killing of some bugs with a biochemical agent? Throw a few antibiotics at the body, and soon you'll be fine.

Yeah, right.

Then there are energy therapies, such as Quantum Techniques (QT), whose holistic applications go beyond the killing of bugs to the identification and removal of toxins of all kinds, including emotional trauma and other environmental poisons that get pent-up in the cells.

Connie Strasheim

QT recognizes that illness isn't simply a product of a few creepy-crawlies, but rather of brokenness, on as many levels as the Empire State building and involving as many layers as the plumpest of onions. Disease is a product of self-hatred and lies we tell ourselves, as well as broken relationships with ourselves, God and others. QT likewise recognizes the role of other environmental toxins in illness, such as pesticides and the plastic food we ingest. Not to mention the bugs, which should be more like an afterthought for some.

This isn't the way we've been taught to think about illness. For any of us to understand Lyme disease on this level would mean doing internet research and consulting God and heeding the intuition within that begs not to be silenced, even though it might be easier to ignore it than to face the demons inside of us.

Yes, a clean case of borrelia burgdorferi may be where it's at for some, but the rest of us will have to get a sharp knife and start peeling the onion, with a willingness to recognize what the mess of chronic illness is often about.

This is what three years of research, my gut and my god have told me. I don't own anyone's truth but my own, but maybe you'll agree I'm on to something here.

And if it's really about bugs and a slew of emotional, spiritual and other environmental toxins, then how does one therapy cover all these bases?

Let me preface my explanation with a science lesson. Quantum Techniques, as other energy healing modalities, believes that illness occurs because of disruptions to and miscommunication within the body's energy field. It also recognizes that cells aren't made up solely of physical matter, because, according to quantum physics, matter is comprised of energy. Yes, you heard right. You are a little bundle of energy (I know, now you are saying, don't I wish!). But it's true.

This energy can be skewed by toxins, whether these are from infections, harmful thought patterns or contaminated food. Consider that all things in existence, all that can be felt and seen and heard, and even that which cannot be observed with the senses but which nonetheless exists, contains a frequency that exerts an influence upon the energy field of the body. That influence is either positive or negative, driving the body towards health or towards disease.

The Chinese have had it right for a zillion years, and we in the West have yet to grasp the concept of energy. When it comes to existence and healing and all things life, energy is a big deal. And what's more, energy can be altered by spoken words.

If you believe in the god of Christianity (as I do), or even if you don't, you might subscribe to the theory that God spoke Creation into existence and that He granted it the power to change the world with words. We humans can build up and tear down, heal and cause disease to ourselves with the words we speak. Quantum Techniques might be thought to harness this belief because it uses spoken codes and affirmations to alter dysfunctional energy patterns in the body and, hence, cellular behavior.

QT also alters the energy of thoughts, which, according to Bruce Lipton in his book, *The Biology of Belief*, have the capacity to alter a person's DNA. Yes, many scientists now think you can alter your genes, for better or worse, by the wicked or loving thoughts you tell yourself.

Because of its holistic applications, Quantum Techniques is worth considering as a primary treatment for Lyme disease and other chronic illnesses. After all, healing from Lyme disease might really mean healing from all kinds of garbage we didn't even know we held inside.

Bioresonance and Similar Energy Therapies

All human and pathogenic cells have electromagnetic frequencies that are measurable and quantifiable, and proponents of energy medicine believe that it's not the biochemistry of pathogens, but rather their energetic properties, that wreak havoc upon us. Illness results when the human body's natural frequencies are disrupted by the frequencies of pathogens, but you can kill these microbes by feeding their reverse energetic imprint back into your body.

This is accomplished with the help of bioresonance devices, which determine which pathogens are causing cellular dysfunction in different organs and systems, by discerning irregular patterns of energy in these areas. Once this information is obtained, the reverse imprint of a particular pathogen's frequency is imprinted into a vial of physiological saline. Then a laser beam is passed through the water and aimed at specific acupuncture points, and the reverse imprint of the pathogen is injected into the body. The energetic imprint then travels along the body's meridians, where it reaches tissues and organs and repels pathogens so that they leave the body.

While its effects on Lyme disease and co-infections are not widely reported, one clinic I spoke with claims a 95% success rate in treating Lyme disease with this therapy. For privacy reasons, I am not including that clinic's information here, but Dr. L. Cowden is one practitioner who employs a similar strategy as part of his protocol for treating Lyme disease patients. The technique he uses is called LED, Laser Energetic Detoxification Therapy. If you do an Internet Google search, you should be able to find the names of other practitioners that perform similar techniques.

Bioresonance therapy is also effective for repelling other foreign substances in the body and therefore can be used to heal many maladies. These include allergies and heavy metal poisoning, which are removed by the same process of bringing the reverse imprint of the allergen or heavy metal into the body. What's more, bioresonance techniques are safe, relatively inexpensive and effective for detecting microorganisms in a manner that western medicine's methods cannot. They are therefore worth investigating as a primary treatment for Lyme disease.

Formulating a Pharmaceutical Antibiotic Plan to Combat Borrelia

Pharmaceutical antibiotics have traditionally been the preferred method of treatment for those suffering from all stages of Lyme disease. While highly effective, especially in the early stages, if you decide to take antibiotics, it is critical that you find an experienced LLMD to set up a treatment plan for you. Relying upon your general practitioner is generally not a good idea, unless he or she has done some research on Lyme disease. It's just too complicated an illness to treat otherwise, and mistakes in treatment are costly, in every sense of the word.

The choice of which antibiotics to take should be tailored to your specific needs, taking into account the severity of your illness, age, ability to tolerate side effects of medications, as well as body composition and co-infections.

If you have chronic Lyme disease (most who are reading this book are likely to be in this stage of illness), then you will need to take two or three different kinds of antibiotics, for at least six months, and more likely, one or more years. For some, an open-ended treatment plan will be necessary in order to attain remission.

The reasons for this are multiple. First, Lyme spirochetes are intelligent organisms that can change their DNA, adapt to antibiotic regimens and morph into a cystic form where they can "hide" in tissue from antibiotics and evade the immune system for years. In the bloodstream, they exist as spiraled bacteria but are also thought to exist in another form that contains no cell-wall, called the "L" form. Their ability to change their composition and form, as well as their expertise in escaping the immune system, require that several different antibiotics be taken for an extended period of time, since no one single drug is capable of killing them in all of their forms, and especially not instantaneously.

Another reason multiple antibiotics are necessary is because Lyme spirochetes are found in both body fluids and tissues, and no single antibiotic is capable of penetrating both areas. Also, according to J. Burrascano, one of the most highly respected and well-known LLMD's, effective antibiotic doses are higher than what is generally recommended by traditional guidelines. This is due to deep tissue penetration by the organisms, their virulence and the difficulty in removing them from the central nervous system. Lyme bacteria disseminate quickly, and their presence can be detected in the CNS as soon as twelve hours after a tick bite, so you can imagine how deeply entrenched they become after months or years in the body!

Your first line of defense against borrelia organisms should include one or two of the following antibiotics: amoxicillin, azithromycin, clarithromycin or doxycycline. If you can tolerate these, then a cyst-targeting drug such as metronidazole or tinidazole should also be added to attack the organism in cystic form.

Oral dosing is preferred; however, if you have been sick for a long time you may want to try IV antibiotics for at least a few months, after which you can switch back to oral medication. Also, make sure that your physician is aware that the method of administration affects an antibiotic's effectiveness and that those that you use in an IV may be different than what you would take orally.

Treatment failures can happen for many reasons, and include, but aren't limited to: your potential allergies to medications, inappropriate dosing by your physician, your ability to adhere to a regimen, and incorrect medication. Keep in mind that antibiotics aren't always compatible with a person's biochemistry and infections, and experimentation with different medications may be necessary. You will also have greater problems eradicating the organism and healing from illness if you have a weak immune system, multiple co-infections or have been sick for a long time.

Finally, antibiotic therapy isn't without risks. Yeast infections and other gastrointestinal problems are common, which in turn affect the rest of the body. Antibiotics are thought by some to weaken the immune system by inhibiting certain enzymatic processes of bacteria and changing the mineral balances of healthy cells. Nonetheless, antibiotics can be powerful and effective for many Lyme disease sufferers and should be taken into consideration as a primary or adjunct therapy for combating Lyme spirochete and other infections.

Herbal and Pharmaceutical Antibiotic Remedies for Babesia, Bartonella and Ehrlichia

Why do co-infections seem to be an afterthought in Lyme disease? Especially when they can be just as, if not more, damaging than borrelia organisms and cause more symptoms than the latter? Whether it's because relatively little is known about co-infections, or because testing methods are even less reliable than those used to diagnose Lyme disease, proper treatment of these is difficult but necessary in order to fully recover from the Lyme disease complex. Following are some widely used herbal and pharmaceutical antibiotics for the treatment of the three most common co-infections. These can be taken separately or combined for greater effectiveness. Most differ from those used to treat borrelia burgdorferi and other strains of Lyme-causing bacteria.

Babesia is the infection most commonly found with borrelia, and artemisia and its derivatives are herbal remedies used to treat it, along with neem and noni fruit. The latter two are especially good to try if you have low ferritin levels, since a certain amount of iron must be present in the body in order for it to effectively utilize artemisia.

Artemisinin is the most widely used derivative of artemisia, and S.H. Buhner, in his book *Healing Lyme*, advocates a 300-500 mg dose for 30-40 days to treat babesia. Other LLMD's and some Lyme disease sufferers have found longer courses, up to six months or more, to be necessary for treating this tenacious parasitic organism, while yet others advocate pulsing the herb. Dr. E. Hesse-Sheehan, D.C., CCN, one of my Lyme disease healthcare practitioners who trained under LLMD Dr. D. Klinghardt, used to recommend that I take doses of up to 1,200 mg of artemisinin daily for a week prior to the full moon, and this proved to be beneficial for me. The choice of which protocol to

Connie Strasheim

follow will depend upon several factors, including your degree of infection, response to treatment and ability to tolerate herxheimer reactions. A similar protocol can be followed for neem and noni.

Also, while artemisinin has typically been the primary derivative of the herb artemisia used to fight babesia, others exist and may be more effective and/or safer than artemisinin and therefore worth trying, especially if you have an active babesia infection that hasn't responded to artemisinin.

Take, for example, artesunate. According to Dr.'s Q and Y. Zhang, M.D., authors of *Lyme Disease and Modern Chinese Medicine*, artesunate is four to five times more active in the body than artemisinin and is just as safe, which makes it potentially more effective than its sibling.

Ozonated rizol oils containing artemisia, such as those produced by Biopure, www.biopureus.com, creatively use the whole herb in a formula that allows deep penetration into tissues. Biopure's rizol oils combine artemisia along with other potent pathogen-killers such as oregano, thyme and garlic.

Other derivatives of artemisia include artemether, arteether, dihydroartemisinin and artemisinic acid. Potentially beneficial and not without risks, they may also be worth using for the treatment of babesia. More information on these can be found in Dr. J. Schaller, M.D.'s book, *Artemisinin, Artesunate, Artemisinic Acid and Other Derivatives of Artemisia Used for Malaria, Babesia and Cancer*.

Finally, as previously mentioned, efficient uptake and utilization of artemisia requires that the body have ample iron stores, as its effectiveness may be compromised in those with low ferritin levels. Supplementing with iron can help, though finding a product that your body will absorb can be challenging, since some iron forms aren't easily uptaken by the body. Dr. Schaller, in his book, *The Diagnosis and Treatment of Babesia*, writes that ferrous heme is an effective form of supplemental iron. Organic organ meats can also be quite beneficial. A friend of mine who suffers from Lyme disease finds that organ meats raise her iron levels more effectively than iron injections!

If you choose pharmaceutical antibiotics to treat babesia, according to Dr. J. Burrascano, M.D., a combination of atovaquone and azithromycin, taken for several months or more, seems to work best for chronic cases. When atovaquone is used alone, babesia sometimes develops resistance to the medication.

Bartonella, the bacteria that produces "cat-scratch" disease, is another vicious infection, and in the co-infected Lyme disease patient, its eradication can be difficult. While many pharmaceutical medications have been shown to be useful against this infection, according to Burrascano, patients tend to fare best with a combination regimen that includes cell-penetrating agents such as erythromycin, plus the antibiotic rifampin. As with babesia, treatment for at least several months is usually required.

In the herbal realm, and according Buhner, Japanese knotweed is beneficial for combating bartonella because it counteracts the angiogenesis actions of the organism by stopping inflammation in the body, which the organism relies upon for its proliferation. It makes a good adjunct to a pharmaceutical antibiotic regimen.

Finally, when compared with bartonella and babesia, ehrlichia seems to be a relatively simple infection to treat. Doxycycline is the antibiotic typically prescribed, although rifampin or another medication may also need to be added. The treatment timeline is often shorter than for bartonella or babesia, with some Lyme disease sufferers requiring only two weeks to a month of antibiotics.

Also, according to Buhner, autumn crocus, or colchicine, is an herb that can be used to treat ehrlichia. His recommendation is to take twenty drops in a tincture for seven days, with a repeat course given after ten days if necessary. This herb is potentially toxic, however, and should be used under the supervision of a knowledgeable practitioner.

Connie Strasheim

Beat Lyme Disease with the Electromagnetic Energy of Rife Machines

Did you know that you can you can harness electromagnetic energy to kill your squirrely spirochetes? Perhaps you've heard of the Rife machine, a device invented in the early 20th century by Dr. Royal Raymond Rife, who discovered that exposing microorganisms to electromagnetic frequencies resulted in their death. If so, you know that his research resulted in the ability to eradicate life-threatening infections, particularly cancer, from the body. Unfortunately, his discoveries were repressed by the powers that be, and knowledge about Rife machines was left up until recently to a privileged few (and the machines are still relatively unknown for the same reason).

The effectiveness of electromagnetic energy for treating Lyme disease was re-discovered approximately fifty years later by Doug MacLean, who built a machine after he inadvertently discovered that this energy had the potential to cure his own Lyme disease. Since then, other machines have been developed and used by the Lyme disease community, with good results. As is the case with most Lyme disease therapies, few people have achieved remission from the use of Rife machines alone; however, in combination with other types of therapy, they can be a powerful primary or adjunct treatment. Results of user polls on the Internet Yahoo! group, Lyme Disease And Rife Machines, (http://www.lymebook.com/resources) have shown Rife machines to be beneficial to varying degrees for almost everyone with Lyme disease.

That said, a lot of machines out there are junk, so it's vital to choose one that has a good track record for treating infections. According to B. Rosner, in his book, *When Antibiotics Fail: Lyme Disease and Rife Machines, with a Critical Evaluation of Leading Alternative Therapies* (www.LymeAndRifeBook.com), there are five types of Rife machines that meet this standard.

The first is the Doug machine, named after Doug MacLean. Extraordinarily powerful, this device is considered by many to have the best track record for treating Lyme disease. It used to be that the Doug was not sold as a complete unit, and some assembly was required. Now, you can purchase pre-assembled machines at www.coilmachines.com. One drawback to the Doug machine is that it only operates on a frequency range of 0-2,200 Hz, and higher frequencies have been found to be useful for treating Lyme disease. It is relatively inexpensive, however, and is great for killing critters.

The second type of machine is an EMEM, or Experimental Electro-Magnetic Machine. While it doesn't have the same track record as the Doug machine, users have found it to be highly effective for treating Lyme disease. Many variations of the EMEM exist, and prices range from $350 to $2,500. This machine is available ready-built, is easy to acquire and use and its frequency ranges up to 10,000 Hz. Some are built to 40,000 Hz, but most effective Lyme disease frequencies have been found to be in the lower ranges. These, and other machines, can be purchased at: www.rifelabs.com.

The next device is an AC Contact Machine, which also requires no skill to set up and is perhaps one of the easiest machines to hook up and operate. It has the highest frequency range of the machines mentioned thus far and even allows for experimentation in the MHz range. Its only drawback might be the cost, which is approximately $2,500. Its effectiveness for treating Lyme disease is similar to that of the EMEM devices. The GB4000 frequency generator and GB-A4 amplifier are preferred by the Lyme disease community as components to look for when shopping for an AC Contact machine.

Another type of device, which doesn't rely upon frequencies to kill organisms but instead utilizes electrical current to electrocute and disable Lyme spirochetes, is the High Power Magnetic Pulser. It was invented by Robb Allen, also a Lyme disease sufferer. Allen found a way to create a device using a DC-pulsed electromagnetic field that would be effective for killing Lyme spirochetes and superior to the well-known Beck and Clark zappers, which have been used to kill other organisms but haven't worked as well for borrelia. This is a great fill-in-the-gap device to frequency machines, as it's thought to be able to kill organisms during a stage in their life cycle that frequency machines cannot. To purchase a magnetic pulser, visit the Internet site: www.highpowermagneticpulser.com.

Of late, more Lyme disease sufferers have been using Resonant Light's Perl machine, which is a $5,000 stellar piece of equipment that utilizes resonant light, an integration of light and sound, to create a signal or frequency that kills microorganisms. The machine is used in hospitals in Canada for treating pain and other disorders. The machine is safe, easy to operate and comes with twenty-four banks of pre-programmed protocols, so you can simply punch in a number, and the machine will run a sequence of frequencies that are effective for your particular infection. One poll on the Internet Yahoo! Lyme-and-Rife group has shown the Perl machine to be more effective than the Doug for treating Lyme disease, although results are yet preliminary. I used a Perl machine for two months and experienced no noticeable herxheimer reactions; however, others have found it to be helpful. For more information on the Perl, check out: www.resonantlight.com.

If you are short on cash, (and even if you aren't!), a good place to look for used Rife equipment is on the Internet site: www.royalrife.com under the "Buy and Sell Used Equipment" tab.

Colloidal Silver, a Tested and True Antimicrobial Remedy

Known to be a successful agent against more than 650 disease-causing microorganisms, including borrelia, colloidal silver has been used throughout the centuries to heal people of all kinds of diseases. Widely used until pharmaceutical antibiotics showed up to shove it aside, renewed interest in colloidal silver has spawned as people learn that antibiotics aren't delivering what they promised, and that colloidal silver as an anti-viral, bacterial, fungal and so forth, has effectively healed many of their maladies. Besides, if taken properly, it won't really turn you into a Willy Wonka blueberry.

Colloidal silver doesn't attack microorganisms directly but instead de-activates enzymes responsible for their multiplication and metabolism. Further, microbes can't mutate into resistant forms, as happens with conventional antibiotics, and while borrelia is smarter than your average bacterial bear, colloidal silver can short-circuit its survival mechanisms to keep it from proliferating.

Many Lyme disease sufferers have used colloidal silver with excellent results and have found it to be useful not only against borrelia but its co-infections, as well. What's more, by purchasing a colloidal silver generator, the stuff can be had for less than a dollar a gallon, which is a bargain over the long run.

In the short run, you'll pay $250 for a decent-quality generator, but then you can have fun in the kitchen and make batches and batches of the sterling stuff, which, unlike your chocolate chip cookies, will last forever and can be kept for long periods of time.

When shopping for a quality colloidal silver generator, don't worry much about how many silver parts per million that it can produce. More important is to find a unit that delivers a uniform product and that doesn't use a constant voltage source, since this tends to screw up silver production. Some generators to try include the Silver Puppy and Silver Gen: www.silverpuppy.com and www.silvergen.com, respectively. If you can't afford to invest in a generator, a good, ready-made colloidal silver product to try is Argentyn 23. Information on this product can be found at: www.naturalimmunogenics.com.

Treating Your Mold and Candida to Heal from Lyme Disease

Since Lyme disease severely compromises immune function, and so many sources of mold and candida exist in our environment, these infections tend to be prolific in those with Lyme disease. I know, as if Lyme disease weren't enough, now you have to contend with these nasties, too?

Chances are, yes, and you may not heal from Lyme disease unless you address these pernicious infections. Don't rely upon symptoms to recognize them, either, as they often mimic those of Lyme disease and discerning them can be difficult. Only a good muscle or visual contrast test or conducting a trial run of treatment as you watch for herxheimer reactions will enable you to determine whether they are a problem. While blood tests can ascertain results, they shouldn't be relied upon as the principal means of diagnosis.

If you often eat leftovers, or anything with gluten or that's packaged in plastic, chances are, you have mold in your body. Don't be fooled; mold can grow on food overnight, even if it is left in the refrigerator. Just because it still tastes okay doesn't mean that it is. I often sauté my leftover rice or packaged nuts to get rid of any mold that might have grown on them overnight and have noticed a reduction in my symptoms by doing so. Your house is another source of the stuff, and discerning whether it has mold can help you to determine whether it also exists in your body. R. Shoemaker's book, *Mold Warriors*, is a good source for learning how to discover and treat mold issues. As you change your diet (and perhaps your home!), consider taking a product such as Tri-Guard Plus: www.oxygennutrition.net., which can help clear mold from the body.

If your diet contains gluten or refined sugar, or you are taking pharmaceutical antibiotics, chances are good you also suffer from an excess of yeast, or candida. This infection can be particularly difficult to eradicate, and a multitude of supplements purport to fix the problem, the majority of which do not work. You must likewise eliminate gluten and sugar if you have a serious candida problem and that means no grains, fruit (except for berries) or simple sugars of any sort. Even dairy products can be a problem. Getting rid of candida is important if you are to recover from Lyme disease. While debate exists over whether it is possible to do this as long as you have Lyme organisms making a mess of the immune system, it is yet important to incorporate an anti-candida protocol into your healing plan if you suspect you suffer from this infection. Cases of Lyme disease that don't respond to treatment are often due to not addressing other infections that are a problem for the body, candida being one of these.

Besides eliminating gluten from your diet, you may also want to try one of the following products:

1. **Diflucan**. This is a highly effective drug for treating yeast. You will need to get your liver enzymes tested regularly if you choose to take this product, as it can be hard on the liver. It is an especially good choice if diet alterations and other supplements don't work.

2. **Tri-Guard Plus**. As mentioned above, this product is also useful for treating mold and is a broad-spectrum antimicrobial, useful for treating parasites, bacteria, viruses, fungi and more. A combination of tea tree oil, grapefruit seed extract and colloidal gold, this product costs around twelve dollars a bottle, which can last a month or more

3. **Cream of tartar**. A rich source of potassium and likewise inexpensive, this product is useful for treating other symptoms of Lyme disease, such as cardiac palpitations and electrolyte deficiencies. It is a good adjunct to the above strategies and may, in some cases, be sufficient for treating candida.

Chapter 2

Detoxification Strategies

The Liver

Cleansing with Beets and Coffee

Okay, so you don't do coffee...coffee enemas, that is. Would you change your mind if I told you that you could get a whole lot of stones and gunk out of your liver with just a few Colombian beans, a carrot, cucumber and a couple of beets?

I know, it's no fun learning how to work with that rubber hose and hot water bottle (plus all the questions from family members who wonder why you are taking that pot of coffee to the bathroom), but hey, isn't a squeaky clean liver worth it? By the way, you're fooling yourself if you think your liver isn't loaded with stones. This is where gallstones come from, too, so before you get your gall bladder removed, try a liver cleanse first, to see if you might also remove the stones from your gall bladder.

Connie Strasheim

The procedure for doing the veggie-coffee enema is as follows:

Juice or eat a couple of beets, a carrot and cucumber approximately two hours prior to the enema. Take some lemon juice and olive oil for greater effect. Don't eat other food as this will diminish results.

Brew two cups of coffee, using two to three tablespoons of organic coffee and filtered water. Don't use it while hot! Add one half-cup to one cup of cool water for every hot cup of brewed coffee.

Lie on your back and flush your colon with water first. Then lie down again. Some enema connoisseurs think it's best to lie on your right side or on your back, while others say it's good to rotate sides. Drain the coffee into your colon, retaining it for ten minutes.

If you don't hear much gurgling and growling activity down in your gut, try using more coffee in the brew next time. I use three to four tablespoons per cup, but for some, this may be too much.

Finally, hover near your best friend john for an hour or two after the enema.

You should feel lighter and even more energetic afterwards. For best results, perform the liver cleanse at least twice weekly, and more often if you are aggressively detoxifying your body.

Another Easygoing Flush

Ridding the liver of toxins is vital for any Lyme disease sufferer's speedy recovery, but not everyone is into coffee enemas or Hulda Clark's amazing but sometimes difficult liver flush (described later). Fortunately, an easier cleanse exists to help rid this magnificent organ of its burden. The effects may not be as dramatic as those produced by Hulda's magic formula, but it can be significant.

The flush is taken from C. Hobbs' book, *Healing with Herbs and Foods*, and uses a preparation of citrus fruit, garlic, ginger, olive oil and herbal tea.

Start by squeezing enough lemons or limes to produce a full, eight-ounce cup of juice. Then add the juice of one or two cloves of garlic, freshly squeezed in a garlic press, and add to that a small amount of freshly grated ginger juice. (Put ginger shreds into your garlic press to get the juice.)

Add one tablespoon of olive oil and then guzzle the mixture, preferably in the morning. Don't eat for an hour following the flush.

Afterwards, Dr. Hobbs recommends drinking two cups of an herbal blend called "Polari Tea," consisting of one part dry fennel, flax, burdock, fenugreek and peppermint, to one-quarter part licorice. Simmer the herbs for twenty minutes, then add peppermint and steep for another ten.

Dr. Hobbs suggests performing this flush daily for ten days, taking a three-day break, and then doing it again for another ten days, repeating twice yearly in the spring and fall. As a Lyme disease sufferer, you may want to do it more or less often, as your body allows.

Unloading the Liver's Burden with Nutrients

"Stop! That's enough, please! Don't give me any more work to do. I can't handle it!"

Can you hear it? I know the voice is muffled (since it lives inside of you), but that doesn't mean it isn't screaming. Yup, it's your liver, protesting in agony at the hordes of detoxification work you've assigned it. Didn't seem like it would be much when you swallowed that herb or popped that pharma-biotic, did it? You didn't know that you'd be asking your poor liver to be the Super Spirochete Sludge Processor, did you?

Fortunately, you can relieve the liver's agony and quiet its clamoring. The easiest way is to pamper it with a coffee enema (as described previously), enhanced by the beet-carrot-cucumber beverage that's given a couple of hours prior to the enema. The enema helps to stimulate the release of toxins from the liver and gall bladder, as do the veggies. Don't worry, the coffee stays in the colon, which means that it won't enter your bloodstream and make you jittery. Enemas aren't difficult, just awkward at first, although when you tell a friend on the phone that you're having a cup of coffee, you might not want to explain how.

A good adjunct to enemas, milk thistle is one of the most powerful herbs for aiding in liver detoxification. When taken alone or in a good combination product such as Liv-52 (www.liv52.com), milk thistle removes toxins while healing the liver.

Another good nutrient to try is glutathione, which is naturally produced by the body and vital for liver detoxification reactions. Sublingual tablets are a practical, convenient way to obtain this nutrient and are thought to be nearly as effective as intravenous glutathione. You can purchase them online or through a compounding pharmacy in the United States such as Lionville Natural Pharmacy, in Lionville, Pennsylvania. (Ph: 877-363-7474). L-methionine (an amino acid) and NAC, N-acetylcysteine (a derivative of the amino acid L-cysteine), when taken together form glutathione, and this is another way to increase stores in the liver. Both nutrients can be purchased in health food stores.

Ensuring a sufficient intake of vitamins and minerals, through foods and supplements, is likewise important, since deficiency in one nutrient causes a cascade of dysfunction in the liver's detoxification mechanisms. Low levels of magnesium, for example, cause reduced levels of glutathione.

Finally, if you are strong enough, consider an intensive liver detoxification strategy, such as that devised by Hulda Clark and described in her book, *The Cure for All Diseases*. For this cleanse, you only need Epsom salts, olive oil, grapefruit juice and a weekend free of activity so that you can rest afterwards.

If you can employ any one of the above strategies, you will nudge your liver back into the direction of becoming the Super Spiro Sludge processor that you need for it to be in order for you to heal from Lyme disease. Then perhaps it will quiet its protests! If it doesn't, consider taking a break from one or more of your Lyme disease treatments so that the poor organ has a chance to rest and unload any backlog of toxins.

The Skin, Kidneys and Lymphatic System

Cleansing the Kidneys with Tea and Herbs

In Lyme disease circles, it seems that few of us think much about how to detoxify the kidneys, focusing instead on the liver and gall bladder. Even the lymphatic system gets more attention. So even though they play a vital role in detoxification and are overworked and underpaid in their job of cleansing the body from toxins produced by Lyme disease and life, the kidneys get shortchanged.

I'll be the first to admit that I've ignored my lima-bean-shaped organs. After all, they haven't complained loudly about all the work I've given them and, like good little soldiers, have performed their job with exceptional efficiency.

Unfortunately, the kidneys tend to stuff their pain, and often it isn't until they are suffering greatly that they clamor to be heard, though damage may have already occurred in the body before any onset of symptoms.

Lower or mid-back pain is one of the kidneys' favorite signals that all isn't right in Kidneyworld. If you are like many Lyme disease sufferers, however, you won't have symptoms of organ dysfunction, but chances are, your kidneys (as most of the body in Lyme disease) are stressed. The quantity of toxins that Lyme disease sufferers must eliminate, along with biochemical dysfunction, practically guarantees this. Fortunately, a few simple remedies can support the kidneys' burden.

These include:

1. **Celery seed tea**. This is prepared by pouring a pint of boiling water over a tablespoonful of freshly ground (or cut) celery seeds. Rich in sodium and potassium, this tea speeds up the clearance of water from the body and toxins from the organs and joints, including the kidneys.

2. **Corn silk tea**. This is thought by some to be the single best herb for increasing urine flow and restoring kidney function.

3. **Watermelon seed tea**. Prepared like celery seed, this tea is a diuretic that speeds up the cleansing and purifying of the kidneys and bladder.

4. **Burbur**. This potent herb detoxifies not only the kidneys but also the liver, lymphatic system and body's matrix.

If you have mid to lower back pain or know that kidney stones are a major problem for you, you may want to try a more in-depth cleanse, such as that described by H. Clark in her book, *The Cure for All Diseases.* Her kidney cleanse recipe can also be found by doing an Internet Google search.

Sweating Out Toxins with Sauna Therapy

When it comes to eliminating toxins from the body, the liver is assigned the brunt of the detoxification process before the toxins receive their discharge papers and are able to make their way out of the body through the colon. Sure, the other organs are involved, but in comparison to the liver, their burden is relatively light.

It doesn't seem fair that one little organ should be responsible for processing the plethora of pathogens and other environmental garbage that Lyme disease generates. The liver's job can be made easier by offering it supports, such as those described earlier in this chapter, but what about removing some of its workload? Is it possible to do this without stopping your Lyme disease treatments?

The answer is yes, but it is thought that the only other way that fat-soluble toxins can leave the body, without having to pass through the liver, is to go through the skin. Nonetheless, it is estimated that up to 30% of the body's toxins can be eliminated this way. While the kidneys aid in detoxifying water-soluble toxins, most Lyme disease toxins fall into the fat-soluble category. Hence the skin, and unless you plan on living in a sweltering climate for a long time, getting the bug muck out via this large organ is best achieved with the help of a sauna.

Acquiring a sauna doesn't have to be expensive. Little canvas ones can be purchased on the Internet on E-Bay: www.ebay.com, for around $100, or you can join your local gym and use the sauna there. Infrared saunas heat the body's core better than most gym saunas, however, and are easier on the cardiovascular system than the more traditional gym saunas.

Choosing to use sauna therapy on a regular basis will accelerate the detoxification process by transferring some of the liver's workload to the skin. Also, the more means that are given to the body to remove toxins, the faster it can pull these from the tissues for processing by the organs, and the more expedient will be a sufferer's recovery.

Helping Traffic on Your Lymphatic Highway with Body Brushing

Did you know that it's estimated that the body contains anywhere from two to ten times more lymphatic fluid than blood? Yet unlike blood, which is propelled by the heart, no organ keeps this fluid moving about the body. Hence, and especially in conditions of illness, the lymphatic system is prone to sluggishness and toxin traffic jams. These prevent it from delivering fluids and nutrients to cells and from picking up toxic waste, including harmful organisms, and shuttling them out of the cells to the lymph nodes.

Finding ways to clear up the congestion can provide healing benefits to the body. One of the least expensive and most efficient methods is to dry brush the skin. Sound bizarre? It did to me, too, and after my first round with the vegetable fiber brush and a bright pink skin rash later, I was ready to chuck the whole idea. As if brushing my hair in

Connie Strasheim

the morning weren't enough of a chore, now I had to brush my body, too?

Fortunately, I didn't toss the brush, and now not only have I become a believer in the benefits of body brushing, but my skin enjoys it, too, as it has ceased to rash up at every BB session.

The benefits of body brushing abound. Foremost is that it accelerates the delivery of nutrients to and the removal of toxins from the cells, which in turn decreases the detoxification burden of the liver, kidneys, lungs and colon. Also, it stimulates the nervous system, blood circulation and lungs, and every organ, ligament, muscle and gland benefits from this. As well, it encourages other systems, including the immune, to operate more efficiently. This can result in a myriad of symptom improvements, including greater energy and cognition, improved digestion and mood, muscular strength and toned skin.

Dry skin brushes can be purchased at your local health food store. Vegetable fiber bristle brushes work best. Instructions for brushing can be found on the Internet, and while simple to perform, the techniques are important to know as they are designed to work in sync with the body's energy pathways, or meridians. Once you get a "handle" on the process, brushing can be accomplished in just five to ten minutes a day.

Additional Strategies

Eliminating Stealth Toxins from Your Diet and Household

September 27, 2004, is my official Lyme disease birthday; or rather, the day when I became incapacitated by Lyme disease, as I suspect I have actually been infected by borrelia for most of my life. Soon after my pseudo-birthday, I chucked my white wine and Cheerios, exchanging these for organic broccoli and herbal tea. I began taking chlorella and doing other toxin removal protocol. The journey continues on to this day, as I continue to find new reasons and new ways to eliminate toxins from my life.

After three years of diligent dedication to garbage removal, you'd think I'd know how to live in an environment free of toxins, but I'm still learning. What I've discovered as of late is that in chronic illness, it's important to take toxins seriously, especially the quiet, sneaky and seemingly unobtrusive ones whose effects you don't perceive.

Such as the mold that's found on nuts and bread packaged in plastic. You don't think nuts have mold just because you don't see green or white fuzzies? Mold is a favorite haunt of any food that's packaged in a plastic bag. Don't despair. You can brown your almonds in the oven before you munch and that will get rid of the mold. Yes, it's a chore, but it's better than that mold having a multiplication-fest in your body.

Then consider dairy. Perhaps you eat organic cow's milk yogurt, and it doesn't cause you symptoms. It may yet be a food your body would rather do without, and whatever isn't beneficial to the cells must be processed as a toxin. The immune system expends energy to get rid of stuff it doesn't need, and in having to divert energy to the waste management process, fewer resources are left to fight infections. Ingesting borderline harmful, or even neutral products, counts.

And forget the little cheats. Even one teeny-weeny bite of a food that the body perceives as an allergen can cause a major inflammatory response that may not manifest as symptoms. It's like carpet-bombing in a war; there's only one bad guy but when the commanders are alerted to his presence, all the troops are sent out. Inflammation, while useful, when overdone can blind the immune system to the presence of pathogens, but it also weakens the body in a multitude of other ways. I once read a statistic that one teaspoon of cane sugar can cause inflammation in the body for up to six hours.

Synthetic household products are likewise damaging. I switched out my personal care items long ago, trading synthetic and harmful L'Oreal, Colgate and the like, for Aubrey Organics and Nature's Gate. I also no longer use commercial laundry soap or cleaning products, preferring Seventh Generation to Tide and Ajax. If you live with

Connie Strasheim

people who insist on using toxic products, humbly ask them to get the stuff, particularly cleaning products, out of the house. Seriously, your recovery may depend upon it.

While you're at it, ask friends and family not to wear artificial fragrances around you. They won't understand why it's a big deal, but you must ask yourself if your health is worth possibly annoying your loved ones a little. You might tell them that products that are difficult for the chronically ill to tolerate are also harmful to those who are relatively healthy. The only difference is that the healthy don't recognize or manifest immediate symptoms.

Once you understand the ramifications of food allergens, as well as the harmful, cell-destroying stuff that goes into non-organic food, cleaning and personal care products, you may never go back to using these again. At the same time, once you are healthier, you may be able to re-incorporate certain foods or relatively safe products back into your diet and life because they will no longer register in your body as allergens.

It feels extreme. It requires extraordinary discipline to stay away from so many toxins, but a sick body needs all the help it can get. Remember, just because somebody successfully marketed a product doesn't mean that it's good for you. Just because everybody eats pizza and wears perfumed lotion doesn't mean that God intended us for to consume and use such things.

The Deleterious Effects of Neurotoxins and How to Remove Them

I tend to blame borrelia for spewing neurotoxins to and fro about the central nervous system, but in reality, the immune system should get part of the blame for being tricked by borrelia to produce its own neurotoxins. Yes, borrelia generates neurotoxins, but it also is a genius at getting the human body to do what it wants for its purposes, and that includes being an accomplice in its garbage production.

For instance, borrelia tricks the microglia, the primary macrophages of the brain, into producing quinolinic acid from tryptophan. While tryptophan is an amino acid needed by the body for neurotransmitter production, quinolinic acid (QUIN) is a potent neurotoxin! As well, borrelia induces the brain to produce ROS (reactive oxygen species) which are, incidentally, made by the body to kill borrelia but which instead function synergistically with QUIN to damage the central nervous system. Destruction to neurons, synaptic connections, brain atrophy and disrupted neurotransmitter production are just some of the ways in which borrelia uses QUIN and ROS to turn the body against itself. I know, you don't want to hear any more. Me neither. Suffice it to say that borrelia sure knows how to hijack the brain's mechanisms.

Fortunately, a number of oral supplements exist to reduce central nervous system damage caused by QUIN and ROS. High-quality chlorella and cilantro remove neurotoxins from the brain. Mucuna bean powder increases neurotransmitter production. Omega-3 and omega-6 fatty acids in your diet help brain cells to regenerate. Japanese knotweed, whose primary constituent is resveratrol, is an herbal antioxidant that neutralizes the effects of ROS and QUIN. Phospholipids prevent ROS damage and help bring other toxin-binders into hard-to-reach areas of brain matter. Zinc prevents hippocampal damage, and melatonin protects neurons, as does lithium orotate. So don't feel bad if you have to take melatonin for sleep, as it will protect your brain while it helps you get your Zzz's!

Using any one of these agents can reduce neurological symptoms of Lyme disease. For best results, you may want to combine a neuronal-protector, such as lithium orotate, with a toxin binder, such as chlorella, as you strive to maintain a diet high in healthy fatty acids and other brain nutrients.

Factors Affecting Your Body's Ability to Remove Toxins

Lyme disease sufferers are not created equal when it comes to toxin susceptibility or the body's ability to detoxify. This may explain why some people progress faster than others in their healing journey and why no single Lyme disease treatment is a panacea. While you may not be able to affect some of the factors that create detoxification problems in the first place, knowing what these factors are can enable you to formulate a plan to make your body's processes more effective.

To start with, men are less prone to the effects of toxins, because they tend to be heavier and with a lower percentage of body fat than women. Since toxins are stored in fat, women get shortchanged. Lifestyle, age, exposure to toxic sources, amount of daily exercise and compromised immune function are other factors that determine detoxification response. Often underestimated is the role of emotional toxins and how unprocessed trauma impacts the body.

Next, certain biochemicals must be present for detoxification, and some Lymefolk are born with, or have acquired, genetic defects that cause them to lack enzymes, hormones or other biochemicals needed for this process. MSH, melanocyte-stimulating hormone and TGF-beta, transforming growth factor, are two of these. Having certain HLA (human leukocyte antigen) haplotypes, which are determined at birth and are part of a person's genetic makeup, can cause compromised detoxification. Testing for all the aforementioned can be performed at local labs such as Quest and LabCorp. Low levels of MSH or TGF, as well as the following HLA DRDQ patterns: 15-6-51, 16-5-51, 1-3-53, 11-5-52b, all indicate that special detoxification measures and/or hormonal supplementation may be required in order to heal the body. Also, sufficient levels of vitamins and minerals must be present in order for the body to utilize these biochemicals.

The next factor affecting detoxification ability regards the liver. The job of detoxification is assigned first and foremost to this organ, and secondly to the skin, kidneys and lungs. The liver is thought to have three times the detoxification capacity as the kidneys and other organs and will break down and remove substances that the others cannot. Since acquired or genetic problems in the liver are other factors affecting detoxification ability, it's a pretty big deal if the liver can't do its job.

Liver detoxification takes place in two phases. In the first, the toxic chemical gets "prepped," so that in the second, a molecule may be added or removed which will enable the toxin to become water-soluble and thereby more easily excreted by the body. More than fifty enzymes under the direction of thirty-five genes are required for phase one to be carried out. Hmmm...kind of makes you wonder what would happen if a person were missing just one of these? It also underscores the importance of taking enough vitamins and minerals so that the myriad of enzymes are fed and fueled up for the task at hand.

Ordinarily, the toxin makeover that a chemical gets in phase one renders it more harmless to the body in phase two, but this isn't always true. Sometimes, reactive chemicals are formed which end up making the toxin scarier and more harmful to the body than it was before it went through phase one. Now, this is no problem if phases one and two are balanced in their activities and the bad chemicals end up being broken down in phase two. But if they are not, the toxin may remain in the body, even uglier now than before the liver a hold of it!

Both phases of liver detoxification require an abundance of nutrients, including fatty and amino acids, vitamins and minerals. Those who are heavily toxic require more of the above than those with a lower toxic burden. Also, protein deficiency is associated with reduced phase one action, and a low-calorie diet affects both phases. One of the processes of phase two, which involves detoxifying drugs, hormones, food additives, heavy metals and neurotransmitters requires more energy than other reactions and will not efficiently take place when a person's energy is low.

With the unique metabolic and detoxification problems that some Lyme disease sufferers have, tweaking the diet is likely to be insufficient for fixing the aforementioned issues, but it can help. Supplementing with enzymes, nutrients, hormones, powerful toxin binders such as cholestyramine or cholestopure may provide greater benefit. In the meantime, understanding the complexities of detoxification can help you to devise new strategies to aid your body in its processes.

Chapter 3

Testing for Infections

How to Determine Whether You Have Lyme Disease and its Co-Infections

You clutch the white IgeneX lab results in your hands, mystified. You have two positive readings for bands 18 and 31 and an indeterminate reading for band 83. Bands 23-25, 34, 39 and 83-93 come up negative. And all the other bands you tested for are somewhat irrelevant.

You have occasional backaches and suffer from OCD, obsessive-compulsive disorder. You also have TMJ (your jaw hurts!). These are your only physical symptoms of illness, so maybe you don't have Lyme disease. After all, many people suffer from such symptoms, and they don't have a tick-borne illness. Not to mention the fact that your physician has told you that there are an excessive number of false positives on test results for Lyme disease, just as there are many false negatives.

How can you be sure? You must treat this illness if you have it, so you're determined to find a way to confirm the results of your test.

Connie Strasheim

According to Dr. J. Schaller and other LLMD's, if you test positive on the IgeneX test to even one of the above-mentioned bands, you have been exposed to a borrelia infection. Whether the infection is active in your body and causing symptoms is a separate issue.

What's more, indeterminate test results for particular bands are really, in the opinion of some LLMD's, weak positives. Lab testers notice a band, but according to test regulations, it must be of a certain size and darkness in order for it to be identified as positive. Hence, they are obligated to state that its presence is uncertain, even if they believe it exists and that the result should be positive.

Let's suppose, however, that you've tested negative with IgeneX, and you have just a couple of symptoms that could be linked to Lyme disease. To ascertain the diagnosis, testing with Central Florida Research (www.centralfloridaresearch.com) is a good idea. In fact, it might be a better lab to start with, because many Lyme disease sufferers don't produce antibodies to infection, and this is what IgeneX and conventional labs measure. Conversely, CFR testing relies upon a positive identification of borrelia in its blood sample.

You can also confirm your diagnosis by performing a CD-57 test through your local lab (fortunately, local labs provide more accurate results with this one), which measures a subset of NK, or killer cells, whose numbers are thought to be low only in those with Lyme disease. A score of less than 60 indicates severe infection, and anything less than approximately 200 means that a borrelia infection is present. Normal results are found in those whose counts are approximately 200 or above. The lower the result, the greater the chance of relapse if a person's treatment regimen is terminated too soon. The only drawback to this test is that it doesn't measure progress in healing, as results can remain unchanged until the infection is well-contained.

Another effective method of testing, if done properly, is applied kinesiology, or muscle testing (we'll talk about this more in the next section). Finding a competent practitioner is important, as many perform its techniques wrong. If you are fortunate enough to be able to find somebody who can do this for you, however, muscle testing is a fast, easy and generally inexpensive way to test for Lyme disease and co-infections.

Bear in mind that ALL testing methods have a margin of error, and there is no Lyme disease test that is 100% accurate. When establishing a diagnosis, the following should also be taken into account:

1. Even if you only have a couple of symptoms, borrelia or other species of Lyme bacteria may be present in your body. Your immune system may simply be containing the development of a more virulent infection. Keep in mind, however, that minor infections can develop into more serious illness and should therefore be treated.

2. Lyme disease is thought by many LLMD's to be an epidemic, but this knowledge remains unacknowledged by the Centers For Disease Control and other organizations, and most physicians ignorant of Lyme disease and testing methods will argue that there are an excessively high number of false positives.

3. Another illness or infection may be the first sign that you have Lyme disease. For instance, you may have been diagnosed, either recently or in the past, with anything from multiple sclerosis to fibromyalgia, chronic fatigue syndrome, candida, herpes, depression and others. Any of these conditions can represent infections or disorders that have occurred in the body due to suppression of the immune system by Lyme disease. They may also be the disguises that Lyme disease wears!

4. Every person, whether healthy or sick, carries antibodies to multiple infections. These infections may or may not be present or active in the body. You may not exhibit symptoms from those that are active, depending upon their severity and the immune system's ability to contain them. If your immune system becomes weakened by stress, however, dormant infections can become active.

Connie Strasheim

5. Whether or not you have tested positive for a borrelia infection on the Central Florida Research or IgeneX test, if you exhibit symptoms of Lyme disease it may be useful to do a treatment and gauge your reaction. This will help determine the accuracy of any test results. Herbal remedies, homeopathy, pharmaceutical antibiotics and Rifing are examples of good therapies to try.

Next, testing for the common co-infections of Lyme disease, particularly babesia, bartonella and ehrlichia, is even more complicated than testing for borrelia, and if you've tested negative with your local lab to these and other important co-infections, chances are, your lab is wrong.

Most Lyme disease sufferers have multiple co-infections and these should not be an afterthought, as they can cause just as many (if not more) symptoms in the body than borrelia. Also, they require separate treatment from borrelia infections, so you'll want to know if you have them.

Central Florida Research and Fry Laboratories located in Arizona, (www.frylaboratories.com), provide the most reliable testing methods for babesia, although they only identify a couple of species, and there are many. Fry Labs also tests for a couple of strains of bartonella, as well as ehrlichia. Yet, it is the most sophisticated and reliable lab in the United States (that I know of) for diagnosing these three common co-infections. As mentioned above, since many species of bartonella and babesia exist, you may also want to seek out a competent muscle-test practitioner to determine whether you have these infections, especially if you test negative with Fry and CFR labs. Muscle testing can determine the presence of infections that cannot be identified by lab tests.

Diagnosis of Lyme disease and co-infections can be challenging, but by performing multiple tests, doing a course of therapy, monitoring symptoms, listening to your intuition and/or asking God for help, you will eventually be able to discover whether you have Lyme disease. The process may take time, but the effort is worthwhile, as untreated, active Lyme disease can develop into a degenerative, debilitating illness.

The Newest Testing Methods: Flow Cytometry and Immunoflourescent Assay

It used to be that Lyme disease sufferers relied solely upon the IgeneX Western blot and the relatively worthless ELISA test to determine whether they had Lyme disease and the more common co-infections of babesia, bartonella and ehrlichia.

As mentioned in the previous section, additional, and perhaps more accurate methods of testing are now being used to test for Lyme disease. These include flow cytometry, from Central Florida Research, and the immunoflourescent assay and stain smear test performed by Fry Laboratories in Arizona.

A flow cytometer is an instrument that identifies bacteria at a rate of 50,000 "events" in the blood per minute. This test can enumerate and quantify borrelia burgdorferi and other strains of borrelia, providing insights into how seriously you are infected with Lyme disease. Unfortunately, as with all Lyme tests, even if you have the disease, you may test negative for the presence of the bacteria, though the incidence is thought to be lower with flow cytometry than with other traditional testing methods. The reason is because this method relies upon a positive identification of the borrelia bacteria, rather than the body's production of antibodies, which is compromised in many Lyme disease sufferers. Other errors in test procedure interpretation are possible but are thought to be volumes lower than with other testing methods. Another benefit to CFC is that some insurance companies, including Medicare, will cover its testing procedures.

Fry Laboratories utilizes the Immunoflourescent assay, which is a serology test, to test for babesia, bartonella and ehrlichia. It identifies both antigens (foreign proteins that are the infectious agents) and antibodies to co-infections in order to detect the presence of infections. As well, it offers a stain smear test, which involves looking at a sample of cells to detect antibodies to other autoimmune illnesses. While many species of bartonella and babesia exist, the lab can only test for babesia microti, bartonella quintana and bartonella henslae, but it is the only lab of its kind in the United States that accurately tests for these infections. Currently, Fry Laboratories is developing a means to test for additional species of co-infections, as there are thought to be many.

All of the aforementioned tests can be purchased together as a package for $495.00.While not covered by most insurance plans, getting one or more tests done by Fry Laboratories may be worth the expense, as your local lab is probably not equipped to accurately test for these difficult-to-detect infections.

How Do You Know if a Supplement Is Right for You? Learning to Muscle Test

You stroll the supplement aisle of your local health food store as the surfeit of products overwhelms you, as it does every week when you go shopping. How do you ever decide what to purchase?

You pause before the collection of iron supplements. Last time you tested, your ferritin levels were low. You decide it's time to get some iron, but which product do you choose? There are just so many brands! After some nail biting, you toss a bottle of Floradix into your cart because you've heard it's most effective.

You continue along but don't get very far before the wheels of your cart stop at the B-vitamin section. You recall that your last saliva cortisol test indicated you have adrenal fatigue, and your health practitioner suggested you take vitamins B-5 and B-6 because these are good for the adrenals. But wait...didn't you read someplace that supplementing with B vitamins throws other nutrients out of whack? You bite your lip and decide to get some anyway. You have no idea which brand works best so you choose a more expensive one, hoping that it will do the job.

As you trudge along, you notice that CO-Q10 is on sale. Your heart has been skipping beats lately, and CO-Q10 is supposed to be good for people with Lyme disease. You're already spending a bundle, but it's important for you to take care of your heart. Of all the organs, this one should not be neglected. So into your cart goes the pricey CO-Q10, and your meandering continues.

Now what was it you came in here for? Oh yeah, your leaky gut! You need to get some acidophilus and so head for the probiotics section. Your eyes glaze over at the myriad of products there. You've heard that most of them are garbage and don't work, so you ask the store clerk and she recommends Jarrow. "It's a favorite of many of our customers," she says. Good enough.

Does this scenario sound familiar? You've probably been through years of guestimating your supplements, haven't you? You purchase things based on what you've read, your physician's opinion, lab test results or your gut feeling. Sometimes, you can tell when a product has helped you to feel better, but at other times you're left wondering.

You may know that just because a supplement purports to fix a problem doesn't mean that it will, and it's not just a matter of choosing quality nutrients. Your biochemistry is unique, just like your fingerprint. As such, just because you know you have an iron deficiency doesn't mean you should take iron. Your body may have bigger reasons for keeping your iron levels low than you are aware of. It may be trying to balance out another problem first, and you will interrupt that process by taking an iron supplement.

For argument's sake, however, let's say that you do need supplemental iron. How can you be sure that the product you choose is going to work with your biochemistry? If the iron is processed in tablet form, for example, you might not have sufficient hydrochloric acid in your gut to break it down. Or your body may need a specific type of iron, but no lab test can tell you which one.

I sometimes wonder how many thousands of dollars I've spent on supplements that haven't worked for me. Was that CO-Q10 or calcium/magnesium absolutely necessary? How could I have known?

While lab tests can be helpful for determining your body's needs, they are often inaccurate and don't tell the whole story about what's going on inside of you.

Fortunately, your body has much wisdom and can tell you exactly what you need, at any given time, through applied kinesiology, or muscle testing, as it is more commonly known. Based on a traditional Chinese concept of internal energy, muscle testing is a non-invasive method of evaluating the body's imbalances and needs. By assessing changes in muscle tension, which are determined either by applying slight pressure to a certain muscle or by moving muscles in a particular direction, substances, infections and other information can be tested for. The person being tested holds the substance or an intention in the mind, such as the thought of a food allergen, as the muscle is moved and its tension evaluated. The substance being tested for may or may not be present; if it is something that the body has come into contact with in the recent past, intentionally focusing upon it may be sufficient for obtaining accurate results. The responses obtained through muscle testing provide information about possible remedies for the body's imbalances, nutritional deficiencies, sensitivities, and so on. Muscle testing can be administered by a trained practitioner, but you can also learn to self-test, although it takes much practice to master! If you can learn its techniques, however, you can more accurately discern which supplements to buy, as well as what infections or imbalances you need to treat.

Quantum Techniques (www.quantumtechniques.com), produces a DVD set, called Truth Techniques I and II, which teaches some of the most accurate, up-to-date muscle testing techniques. Again, these take practice to master, but with time, many people can learn how to test themselves. By applying the techniques every time you go shopping, you can be empowered to choose products that your body needs, while avoiding the ones that it doesn't need.

Just because a supplement claims to fix a certain problem in your body, doesn't mean that it will. Just because a famous healthcare practitioner suggests it or you've read about its benefits on several Internet Yahoo! Groups, doesn't mean you should run out and buy it. Learn to muscle test yourself. It's the only way to know for certain, short of trying out a product, whether it will work for you.

Chapter 4

Hormone Balance

The Healing Power and Dangerous Potential of Supplemental Cortisol

Supporting the adrenal glands while combating Lyme disease and other infections may be important for recovery, since the immune system depends heavily upon cortisol, a primary steroid hormone produced by the adrenal glands, to work its healing magic upon the body. Supplemental cortisol can aid in the recovery process when the body is not able to synthesize enough of its own hormone, but much controversy surrounds its use, and with good reason.

Moderate and high doses of natural and synthetic cortisol, found in products like Isocort or Cortef, have been known to send the adrenals into shutdown mode for good, and especially when the hormone is given every day. They are also thought to confuse the body's own cortisol production processes. They can cause inflammation, suppression of the immune system and proliferation of Lyme bacteria. Another problem is that regulation of any supplemental hormone is dependent upon a physician's discernment and subjective lab results rather than the wisdom of one's internal mechanisms. Until recently, physicians have not known how much natural cortisol the body produces and therefore have had a tendency to prescribe either too much or random amounts of cortisol, which has had deleterious effects upon patients. This may be part of the reason why cortisol has gotten a bad rap and had disastrous effects upon its users.

What's more, those who have taken hydrocortisone, prednisone or a similar steroid and suffered damage to their bodies, know that these supplements can indeed be harmful.

Some schools of thought, however, such as that found on the website: www.stopthethyroidmadness.com and in Dr. Jefferies, M.D.'s, book, *Safe Uses of Cortisol*, teach that low to moderate doses of cortisol (at least more moderate than those traditionally prescribed!) pose little danger of adrenal shutdown. Jefferies contends that cortisol can actually aid the immune system rather than suppress it, as, ironically, one of cortisol's functions is to inform the body not to overdo inflammation when it is under physiological stress. Too much inflammation causes cellular destruction and blinds the immune system to the presence of the Lyme bacteria, and by reducing the body's inflammatory response, cortisol can help to minimize cellular damage and eradicate borrelia infections.

Also, the functions of cortisol produced naturally by the body are life-giving. You would die without this steroid hormone, and any deficiency stresses the body, just as does any excess.

Hence, cortisol is both inflammatory and anti-inflammatory. It can heal or harm, and for this reason it is a hormone that deserves our utmost respect. Extreme care must be taken when it is artificially administered to the cortisol-deficient Lyme disease sufferer. I personally know one Lyme disease sufferer who would have died without synthetic cortisol, and he is now in remission. I also know a couple of others whose healing has been hindered by synthetic cortisol, due to immune system suppression and inflammation. I don't know if these people were prescribed inappropriate doses, or if their bodies simply reacted badly to the steroid hormone.

Personally, I have found that five milligrams of Isocort, an adrenal glandular formula containing small doses of active cortisol from New Zealand sheep, gave my body a much-needed boost during months when my adrenal fatigue was so bad I couldn't breathe or stand up for more than two minutes. After several months, its effectiveness waned. I don't know if this was due to my body sensing the presence of the hormone and shutting down its own cortisol production, or if it stopped working for some other reason.

However, some people take natural or synthetic cortisol for years and experience continued positive results.

If you are suffering symptoms of severe adrenal fatigue, supplemental cortisol might be worth considering, as this powerful hormone, when administered properly, can accelerate healing. Indeed, for some, it may mean the difference between living a functional life or being tied to the sofa. Keep in mind, however, that using cortisol to treat Lyme disease is highly controversial and some of the best LLMD's in the country strongly advise against its use due to the risk of dangerous immuno-suppression that can lead to proliferation and increased severity of the Lyme disease infection.

The Fussy Thyroid and How to Fix It

Many people with Lyme disease suffer hyperthyroidism, or more commonly, hypothyroidism. In the first scenario, the thyroid produces too much hormone; in the second, not enough. Thyroid hormone supplementation can help balance this little gland, so that you aren't a hyper hare plugged into a socket or a fog-brained achy blob on the couch. Trying to find an optimal thyroid "food" that your body will respond to, as well as an appropriate dosage, can be challenging, but is a worthwhile endeavor that will help you to feel your best as you treat Lyme disease.

Some synthetic thyroid supplements are made from T4 thyroid hormone, and these rely upon the body to convert T4 into T3, which is the primary thyroid hormone that the body utilizes for its biochemical

Connie Strasheim

purposes. The problem with T4 synthetics is that folks with Lyme disease or CFIDS (Chronic Fatigue and Immune Dysfunction Syndrome) often convert T4 into an unusable form of T3, termed "reverse T3," and hence cannot utilize synthetic T4 hormone. A better choice would be pure, bioidentical T3, which can be obtained at compounding pharmacies, or another form of T3 called Armour Thyroid made from bovine thyroid gland. If ingesting another animal's organs gives you the heebie-jeebies, then stick with bioidentical, synthetic T3.

If your hypo or hyperthyroidism isn't severe, it's worthwhile to consider iodine supplementation before hormone replacement therapy, since the body synthesizes thyroid hormones from iodine. This is a better way to help it along, as the body can decide for itself what it needs to make thyroid hormones, whereas with hormone replacement, it doesn't have much choice but to swallow the stuff. If your body isn't capable of synthesizing thyroid hormone from iodine, however, hormone replacement therapy may be a necessity.

Persevere...there are several supplemental options for balancing the thyroid, and the optimal choice will be different for everyone.

Causes of, and Solutions for, Hypothalamic-Pituitary-Adrenal Foul-Ups

The fact that multiple causes exist for hypothalamic-pituitary-adrenal (HPA) dysfunction in Lyme disease drives me up a jagged wall. How much better I'd feel if I could only figure out how to make my endocrine system function properly! Fortunately, I do have a few insights to offer you in the area of HPA dysfunction that have helped me to control my haywire hormones and which may help you, too.

To begin with, endocrine foul-ups can be caused by, among other factors: pituitary insufficiency, central inhibition of the hypothalamus (the former often caused by the latter), and adrenal fatigue caused by trauma and/or Lyme neurotoxins that bind to receptor sites on the HPA axis. That means that bug garbage sticks to places on your pituitary, thyroid and adrenal glands and screws up hormone operations there.

HPA dysfunction may also occur as a result of nutritional deficiencies. Where digestive and other processes are inefficient, the entire endocrine system will be short on resources for building and utilizing hormones. Some Lyme disease sufferers have problems digesting protein, which is crucial for building biochemicals, and no raw materials means no finished product.

The thyroid and adrenals are called upon to work overtime when faced with illness, and problems may result from too many demands being placed upon these poor little glands. Further, other biochemical dysfunction caused by Lyme disease has a domino effect on the body, impacting the endocrine system. Insomnia, for example, can be a cause or result of hypothalamic suppression, which then affects the entire HPA-axis.

Emotional stress caused by borrelia neurotoxins or current or past trauma is likewise harmful, because anger, depression and anxiety induce the adrenal glands to secrete excess levels of adrenaline and cortisol. Over the long haul, this burns them out so that they are unable to function properly.

To solve any of the above problems, try taking supplements that feed these glands, such as iodine and adrenal glandular formulas. An adequate supply of vitamins and minerals is also important. The adrenals, in particular, need vitamins C, B5 and B6. Herbs such as licorice and Siberian ginseng can likewise be helpful. In cases of severe HPA dysfunction, support the thyroid and adrenals with natural hormones such as cortisol, DHEA and T3 (thyroid).

Taking a high-quality neurotoxin binder, such as chlorella, apple pectin or mucuna bean powder will remove toxins from HPA receptor sites and can help to restore proper function to the endocrine system.

Next, eating balanced meals that include sufficient amounts of protein and essential fatty acids (as well as enzymes to help digest them) will help rebuild and replenish deficient hormones.

Finally, keeping stress to a minimum and performing therapies to heal emotional trauma is vital for recovery from endocrine foul-ups, as every time the body is subject to the sensation of fear, cortisol and adrenaline are released into the bloodstream. When constant and prolonged, this biochemical phenomenon taxes the body. While you may struggle to eliminate anxiety from your life, even small changes in your mental outlook or life's circumstances can give your endocrine system a boost in ways you hadn't thought possible.

Optimizing Insulin, Adrenaline and Cortisol Function and Production

Why do we Lyme disease sufferers pay so much attention to optimizing thyroid function?

Sure, it plays a vital role in metabolism, but did you know that its function is governed by a more important hormone, cortisol? Along with insulin and adrenaline, cortisol governs the activity of all other hormones in the body. According to Dr. Schwarzbein, author of *The Schwarzbein Principle II,* by balancing these three major hormones, the body can get a better grip on the minor ones, such as DHEA, thyroid, testosterone and estrogen. And anything we can do to keep our hormones in order will strengthen our immune system in the battle against Lyme disease!

Basically, and in concert with other hormones, cortisol and adrenaline sustain life by regulating blood pressure and blood sugar, and mobilizing energy, by metabolizing biochemicals so that you can put them to use for all of your body's functions. Insulin, in a broad sense, does the opposite by helping the body to rebuild biochemicals from food. It also prevents you from using up too many biochemicals if you don't get enough food.

Eating proper amounts of protein and carbohydrates is the easiest and most important way to balance the Big Three. According to Dr. Schwarzbein, when you eat too many carbohydrates and not enough protein at mealtimes, this raises insulin levels too high in your body, as does eating too much food in one sitting. Conversely, eating too much protein and not enough carbohydrates stimulates the production of excess adrenaline and cortisol, as does eating a protein by itself or skipping meals (and especially the latter).

If you have Lyme disease, your poor adrenal glands are working overtime to heal your body and will resent you even more if they have to contend with the extra work of secreting excess adrenaline and cortisol every time you graze improperly. Furthermore, according to Dr. Schwarzbein, excess levels of these hormones circulating in the bloodstream create a multitude of imbalances in the body and cause you to use up your structural and functional biochemicals faster than you can rebuild them. These biochemicals are needed for your healing. Perhaps you care for your adrenals by avoiding caffeine, sugar and stress, or maybe you take adrenal glandular formulas and herbs. So how about relieving them of their digestive burden, too?

On the other hand, too much insulin from excessive carbohydrate intake causes too much biochemical production, and you'll have more sugar for energy and rebuilding your parts than your body knows what to do with. And what does your body do with that extra sugar? You guessed it. It puts it into storage for a rainy day that will probably never come. The long-term effects of an over-consumption of carbohydrates include weight gain, hypertension, abnormal cholesterol and arteriosclerosis.

If you are like me, you'll be tempted to stay away from certain complex carbohydrates, such as brown rice and potatoes, as any excess of sugar is thought to feed borrelia. However, consider that a diet that goes light on the starchy veggies, legumes and grains will also tend to raise your cortisol and adrenaline levels. You may feel better when you stay away from starchy carbohydrates (after all, having excess cortisol and adrenaline floating around in your body keeps your energy higher), and you're probably allergic to most grains, but try to stick a few of

Connie Strasheim

these food types back into your diet. Yes, it is important to stay away from foods that feed your infections, but this should be only one consideration when formulating a diet plan.

Also, while it is true that some Lyme disease sufferers have trouble metabolizing protein, the body needs it in order to make hormones and other biochemicals. If you suffer from this problem, take protein frequently in small amounts, along with a small carbohydrate snack.

Using vitamin, herbal and glandular supplements can also support the production and proper use of these hormones. Through muscle testing, which provides more accurate results than standard blood, saliva or urine tests, you can ascertain which hormones or supplements your body needs. Bear in mind that the latter tests only measure circulating levels of hormones, without taking into account whether your body is actually using them. They ignore your unique biochemistry and other factors which affect whether a supplement would be beneficial for you. Muscle tests are better because they tell you what your body actually needs, all things considered.

Managing stress is also a crucial step for optimizing hormone function, especially adrenaline and cortisol, as these hormones are quickly depleted under conditions of stress, whether physiological, chemical, nutritional, or hormonal. Living in a state of fear, in particular, releases huge amounts of cortisol and adrenaline into the bloodstream, which weakens the immune system.

So relax, eat balanced portions of protein and complex carbohydrates and muscle-test to determine whether hormonal or other nutritional supplements can normalize your hormones' operations for better health.

The Link Between Adrenal Fatigue and Hypothyroidism and Why It Matters

Hypothyroidism and adrenal fatigue are common in Lyme disease sufferers, but did you know that adrenal fatigue is often the reason for hypothyroidism? Yet it's usually treatment of the latter that is given greater attention.

Many Lyme disease sufferers produce insufficient quantities of cortisol, a primary adrenal hormone that is required for thyroid hormone uptake into cells. If you're feeding your thyroid with synthetic or natural thyroid hormone, you may yet remain hypothyroid, because in the absence of sufficient cortisol, you will have excess thyroid hormone floating around in your bloodstream that gets unused by the body.

By supporting the adrenal glands so that cortisol production is increased, some Lyme disease sufferers have found that they are able to reduce how much thyroid hormone they take. This is fantastic news for anyone who is frustrated by a sluggish thyroid that stubbornly refuses to respond to increased dosages of thyroid hormone.

Chapter 5

Adjunct Lyme Disease Treatments

Nutrients for Immune Function

Fixing a Broken Lyme Heart with Herbal Remedies and Other
Nutrients

No pun intended here. Lyme is hard on the heart, in a number of
ways. Hypercoagulation, a thickening of the blood due to borrelia's
bacterial schemes, means that the heart has to work harder to pump
blood. The presence of borrelia in this organ causes blood pressure
foul-ups, angina, tachycardia and other autonomic nervous system
dysfunction. Nutrient deficiencies caused by Lyme disease mean that
the heart doesn't get what it needs for proper functioning and
biochemical repair. Protecting this precious organ and ensuring that it
gets an adequate supply of nutrients can ameliorate cardiac and other
symptoms and safeguard it against damage.

To begin with, Lyme disease sufferers often overlook the importance
of treating hypercoagulation. When the blood is too thick, the heart
strains to pump it throughout the body, and nutrients and oxygen

don't reach the cells as easily. Treatment with natural enzymes and anti-coagulants such as Rechts-Regulat, Nattokinase and Wobenzyme or the prescription drug heparin can alleviate this problem.

Also, most Lyme sufferers are deficient in Coenzyme-Q10, a substance normally found in abundance in the heart and which is involved in energy production. Supplementing with a quality CO-Q10 product ensures the heart's energy furnace is supplied with ample fuel for its active, 24/7 job.

Next, hawthorn can be helpful for treating autonomic nervous system dysfunction. This remarkable herb normalizes blood pressure, raising or lowering it as needed, as it regulates heart rhythm, increasing or slowing it as the body dictates. It eliminates arrhythmia's and creates efficient contractions of the heart, so that it beats more powerfully. Ensuring an adequate intake of the macro-minerals magnesium, potassium and calcium also helps to regulate and normalize heart rhythms.

Khella is another stellar heart herb. It dilates coronary arteries, increasing the heart's blood supply. A couple of other herbs, andrographis and Japanese knotweed, which are used for treatment of other conditions in Lyme disease, are also cardio-protective.

You don't need to suffer with a broken heart. Solutions exist to help you reduce your cardiac symptoms so that your heart will beat with power and the joy of health.

Cordyceps Mushrooms for Energy, Immune Support, and More

If cordyceps weren't so pricey, I'd be popping these shrooms like candy. And the truly worthwhile ones cost precious coin. So what's so great about cordyceps?

This remarkable mushroom, cultivated in China, is known for providing a myriad of benefits to Lyme disease sufferers. Besides increasing energy and blood flow to the heart, it lowers LDL's (low-density lipoproteins), combats arteriosclerosis and helps to normalize heart arrhythmia's.

By activating NK-cell and macrophage activity, as well as enhancing T-cell activity, it's a great friend to the immune system. Its effects upon NK-cell activity are especially useful for Lyme disease sufferers, since one of borrelia's proliferation strategies is to dramatically reduce NK-cell counts.

Cordyceps also sedates the central nervous system, which is great news for those who suffer from anxiety, hyperactivity and other neurological problems caused by Lyme disease.

Further, it increases red and white blood cell, platelet and lymph cell counts. Considering that Lyme and co-infections gobble up and destroy these cells, replacing them is vital for proper biochemical function.

Finally, because cordyceps is anti-asthmatic and dilates the lungs' airways, it can be beneficial for those with babesia and adrenal fatigue since both conditions cause breathing problems.

Treating Multiple Symptoms with Japanese Knotweed

Stephen H. Buhner is a master herbalist who has made remarkable discoveries about how to treat Lyme disease with herbs. If I ever have the pleasure of meeting him, I will toss gratitude flowers at his feet for having introduced me to Japanese knotweed, or polygonum cuspida-tum, an herb that has more uses in Lyme disease than I have fingers on my hands. For the sake of space and your patience, I'll enumerate only the most important ones here.

By reducing inflammation, Japanese knotweed helps the body to combat infections, since inflammation blinds the immune system to the presence of borrelia, bartonella and other pathogens. Its anti-inflammatory properties, which are due in part to resveratrol and trans-resveratrol, two important constituents of the herb, are also beneficial for treating arthritis.

Connie Strasheim

Next, Japanese knotweed is an anti-everything, capable of killing bacteria, fungi, viruses and every pathogen under the moon. It is known to kill some varieties of spirochetes, and that may include borrelia burgdorferi. It is a powerful immunomodulator, raising immune function when necessary and lowering it when it's in over-drive.

Further, Japanese knotweed protects the body against neurotoxin damage and reduces central nervous system symptoms. It increases blood flow and hence the transport of treatments to hard-to-reach areas of the body, such as the eyes, heart, skin and joints, and is an antioxidant that helps to reduce herxheimer reactions. Finally, it protects the heart and helps to reduce symptoms of Lyme carditis.

I could go on and on about the benefits of Japanese knotweed, but I'll finish my rave here with a recommendation for a good source of the herb, which is found at Supplemental Health Formulations, LLC.: www.shfnatural.com, or 1st Chinese Herbs, www.1stchineseherbs.com.

Enzymes and other Solutions for Thick Blood

Triggering hypercoagulation, or an excess clotting of the blood, is a favorite tactic of Borrelia and the Co-infection Gang for blocking the body's cells from receiving the nutrients they need for proper function. Many Lyme disease sufferers are unaware that they have this some-times dangerous condition, whereby the blood becomes too thick as a result of fibrin being deposited into blood vessels, resulting in reduced blood flow to capillaries so that less oxygen and fewer nutrients make it to the cells. Fibrin is normally produced in the last stages of the blood clotting process, but in folks with CFS, fibromyalgia and Lyme disease, the process is haphazard.

Borrelia also uses this strategy to protect itself from antibiotics and other anti-bug warfare, as fibrin serves as a nice, cozy fortress for it to hide from anti-spirochetal drugs.

The blood is further affected by circulating protein debris, comprised of immune complexes (antibody-antigen pairs) that are created when the immune system gets into a fight with borrelia. These compromise the body's functioning by putting the immune system into hyper-stimulus and hyper-inflammation mode. This protein debris likewise contributes to hypercoagulation.

Traditional medicine treats these problems with heparin, but who wants to inject a needle into their gut twice a day and get blood tests drawn every week? Some natural enzymatic products, such as Nattokinase, Wobenzym and Rechts-Regulat, are good alternatives to heparin. Not only do they thin the blood, but they also cleanse it of circulating immune complexes, which allows the immune system to reduce its inflammatory attack upon the body, as it no longer perceives the presence of protein globs in the blood. Also, as the blood gets a bath, oxygen and nutrients flow more freely to the cells and circulation is improved.

Other remedies, such as Vitamin E and omega-3 fatty acids, can aid in thinning the blood when other products become inconvenient or cost-prohibitive or, more often, when additional support is required. Ironically, when too many omega 6's are present in the diet, blood clotting is fostered. By ensuring a 1-3 ratio of omega 3 to omega-6 fatty acids, the body will better balance its blood-clotting activity. Most people get too much Omega 6 in their diets, so adding an Omega 3 supplement may be beneficial.

If you are a victim of borrelia's blood-thickening plot, it's important to treat hypercoagulation. Not only so that your deprived organs get the nutrients they need, but also because thick blood brings other agony to the body, including a higher risk of clots and a heart that has to work harder to pump blood.

Super Siberian Ginseng for Mood, Stamina and Immune Function

I wonder if God allowed Siberian ginseng, (a.k.a. eleutherococcus senticosus), to flourish in Russia because He knew its people would need something powerful to withstand their harsh, dark and cold

Connie Strasheim

living conditions. This may be a silly hypothesis on my part, but what I'm about to tell you about the herb is not.

In Lyme disease, Siberian ginseng increases one's capacity to withstand adverse conditions by increasing stamina and mental alertness, at the same time that it reduces depression and mood swings.

Fatigued adrenals crave ginseng. It acts as a tonic to the glands, rejuvenating and revitalizing them, which brings positive effects to the rest of the body.

Next, the immune system gets a helping hand from ginseng, as the herb increases production of natural killer and T-lymphocyte cells, which tend to be deficient in Lyme disease sufferers.

Stumbling adrenals may benefit from the powerful 2:1 Russian formulation by Herb Pharm:, www.herb-pharm.com, though weaker concoctions may be preferred by hyperactive souls. Siberian ginseng isn't an herb to take continuously. Breaks must be given every couple of months, for a few weeks at a time, especially for stronger formulations.

If you suffer from chronic fatigue, hypothyroidism, adrenal fatigue, mood swings and/or depression, lack of stamina, low immune function and brain fog, just to name a few, eleutherococcus senticosus may be worth considering as an important adjunct treatment for Lyme disease.

Natural Anti-Inflammatory Treatments

Borrelia is a master at coaxing the immune system into blinding itself with inflammation. This is so that it can't see and attack the crafty bacteria. Borrelia does this strategically, because inflammation enables its proliferation and survival.

Happily, options exist for reducing inflammation. Vitamin C and essential fatty acids (such as fish and flaxseed oil) rank at the top of the list, along with proteolytic enzymes.

Bromelain, or pineapple enzyme, is one of the most beneficial of these and has the added benefit of breaking down fibrin and reducing hypercoagulation, a common condition in Lyme disease.

Herbs aplenty also exist for separating Inflammation from its pal Borrelia. Turmeric is one. I personally love seasoning my meats and veggies with this tasty Indian spice. Olive leaf extract is also useful, and it has the added benefit of being a powerful anti-microbial agent. Boswellia, echinacea, ginger, goldenseal, pau d' arco and red clover are others to try.

Eating foods high in flavonoids, which are super anti-oxidants, is another useful strategy for severing the Borrelia-Inflammation relationship. Spinach and berries are examples of good sources for this.

So season your meat with turmeric, make yourself some pau d'arco tea, have a bit of pineapple for breakfast or find other creative ways to incorporate anti-inflammatories into your diet. In doing so, you'll give your immune system sharper eyes for recognizing borrelia.

Enhancing Immune Cell Production with Transfer Factor, Glutathione and More

An immune system compromised by Lyme disease needs all the help it can get to fight borrelia and the party of pathogens it invites into the body. One way to keep it kicking is through the aid of oral supplements designed to enhance the effects of different types of immune cells.

First, Lyme disease tends to diminish a subset of NK, or natural killer cells, called CD-57. NK cells are known for their amazing ability to recognize and quickly destroy viruses, cancer and other pathogenic cells upon contact. Decreased numbers of NK cells are associated with chronic infection and immune dysfunction. One way to increase them is by transferring immunity from a healthy host animal via colostrum (mother's first milk after birth) which is loaded with nutrients. This

Connie Strasheim

colostrum is appropriately called transfer factor. 4 Life Research makes a good transfer factor product that can be purchased online at: www.4tf.com. Cordyceps mushroom, in addition to being an energy enhancer, also boosts NK-cell production.

Other immune cells involved in gobbling up microbes are macrophages, whose name literally means "big eater." These cells swallow foreign proteins whole, and, once the proteins are engulfed, the cells destroy or neutralize them. They are the vacuum cleaners of the immune system and scarf down any tissue that isn't needed by the body. To stimulate this class of immune cells, try Beta-1, 3-Glucan, found in most health food stores. This is a simple sugar derived from the cell wall of a type of yeast, though it is thought not to provoke reactions in those who have yeast allergies.

Supporting the thymus can also be helpful for enhancing immune cell production. This little gland sits behind the sternum in the chest, and its principal task is to release proteins that stimulate white blood cells. It acts like a thermostat, regulating the release of immune cells for the body's use. Taking thymus gland from a healthy cow supports optimal function of this gland. ProBoost is a good bovine product to try. You can purchase it online at: www.immunesupport.com/pro_boost.htm, as well as on other Internet sites.

Finally, L-glutathione is a superstar amino acid complex that plays an important role in immune function. In addition to being a free-radical scavenger, it supports the activity of a group of white blood cells called lymphocytes (the key players in the body's immune response, which are comprised of several subtypes, including antibodies). Without glutathione, lymphocytes can't do their job properly.

Glutathione is naturally produced in the liver, and because most Lyme disease sufferers have liver problems, the body may not have an adequate supply to offer the immune system. Supplemental glutathione can help remedy this problem and can be taken intravenously, sublingually, intramuscularly or orally. The greatest combination of convenience and effectiveness might be realized, however, when glutathione is taken in sublingual form. Another option is to take products containing glutathione precursors, which include glutamic acid, cysteine and glycine. Immunocal, www.immunocal.com, is one product that contains all three of these amino acids.

Boosting the Body with Stem Cell Enhancers

Lyme disease is vicious in its ability to destroy cells, but stem-cell enhancing products can help the body to rebuild itself more quickly and fix the mess that borrelia has left behind. Stem cells, found naturally in the human body, maintain and repair the tissue in which they are found by becoming whatever type of cell the body happens to need, whether that be a liver, heart or kidney cell. Reservoirs of stem cells are found in certain organs and tissues, and stem cell enhancing supplements are designed to promote their release from these tissues so that parts of the body become more quickly regenerated and/or repaired.

One effective product, a botanical extract called StemEnhance by Stem Tech Health Sciences (www.stemtechwellness.com), releases stem cells from bone marrow, where they circulate and are utilized according to the body's needs. Studies have shown stem cell circulation in the body to be increased by up to 30% with this product.

Of late, a handful of Lyme disease sufferers have been using stem cell enhancers and have experienced increased energy, as well as a reduction in other symptoms. Stem cells have been used in a variety of illnesses, including cancer, with good results. While data on its long-term effects as a helpful healing adjunct for Lyme disease is unknown, the preliminary results of its use are encouraging.

The true test of this therapy's effectiveness may reside in its continual ability to render more effective the body's use of its own stem cells, as how stem cell products accomplish this is somewhat of a mystery.

Increasing Iron Stores to Combat Babesia

Lyme disease and babesia are partners in crime. It seems no accident that the two infections are often found together. Babesia starves the body of oxygen by destroying red blood cells which carry oxygen to other cells. Borrelia thrives in this anaerobic environment, and consequently, the body has a more difficult time fighting Lyme disease than if it simply had to contend with just one infection.

Increasing your iron intake can help remedy this problem, since the body uses iron to create hemoglobin, the substance in red blood cells that carries oxygen. Also, as previously mentioned, the body requires that a certain amount of ferritin (iron stores) be present in order for it to utilize artemisinin, a commonly prescribed herb to treat babesia, so taking iron can be important if you choose to treat with artemisinin.

Also, as mentioned earlier, iron is a finicky mineral that can be difficult for the body to uptake, so taking iron injections may be necessary. However, it may be worth it to first try ferrous heme or organic organ meats, as these are thought to be highly absorbable oral forms of iron. If you choose to take an oral supplement, have some Vitamin C or orange juice along with it to double its absorption. It is also important not to take iron at the same time that you take calcium or magnesium, as doing so reduces its absorption.

Certain B vitamins are necessary for iron uptake and utilization, especially B-12, B-1 and B-6, so choose an iron supplement that includes these vitamins, or consider adding foods to your diet that contain high levels of B-vitamins. Some LLMD's believe most Lyme disease sufferers to be deficient in vitamin B-12, and injections may also be the only effective way to raise the body's level of this vitamin.

Finally, if you have Lyme disease but have not been diagnosed with babesia, yet have low ferritin levels, suspect that the latter infection may nonetheless be present.

Supplemental Oxygen for Life and Lyme

Borrelia and oxygen are fierce enemies. Borrelia thrives in an anaerobic environment, where it deprives the body of oxygen so that it cannot fight infection.

All biochemical processes depend upon oxygen for life, and two-thirds of the body's oxygen consumption is used to produce energy for cells. Without this energy, cellular dysfunction occurs, resulting in innumerable problems for the body.

Lyme disease sufferers are typically oxygen-starved, and this is part of the reason for fatigue and other symptoms. In the absence of oxygen, detoxification processes become inefficient, digestion is poor, white blood cell function is slowed, red blood cells clump and cellular metabolism becomes dysfunctional. Basically, nothing works right.

Fortunately, Lyme disease sufferers can increase oxygen in the body, and not just through hyperbaric oxygen chambers, which can be cost-prohibitive.

The simplest way is through aerobic exercise and deep breathing routines. Keeping stress to a minimum, ensuring an adequate intake of minerals and eating balanced meals can also help, as overeating, stress and mineral deficiencies increase the body's need for oxygen. Also, increasing your intake of antioxidants helps the body to utilize oxygen more efficiently.

Avoid carbon monoxide, such as that from vehicle exhaust and gas stoves, since this chemical reduces the oxygen-carrying capacity of the blood. Also, keep a few green plants around the house, as these absorb carbon monoxide.

If you have a few more dollars, consider obtaining an ozone generator as another potent source of oxygen. Ozone is often used topically or as a rectal infusion, and an ozone bath is thought to provide as much benefit as a hyperbaric oxygen chamber. You can also ozonate your drinking water. Ozone also provides many other benefits to Lyme disease sufferers, so investment in an ozone generator may be worth the expense.

Other Adjunct Healing Strategies

<u>Dying for Some zzz's: Causes of, and Solutions for, Insomnia</u>

It's midnight, and you've been lying awake for two hours, your thoughts on fast forward as you toss and turn like a vegetable kabob over a spit. You get up to take yet another potty break, toss and turn some more, then head to the kitchen for a 1:00 A.M. yogurt. You go back to bed and fall into a twilight slumber filled with absurd dreams of your ex. You awaken at 5:00 A.M., exhausted. You try to go back to sleep, but do the shish kabob thing again until 8:00 A.M. at which time you fall into another quasi-slumber until sleep apnea and feeling suffocated in your dreams finally compels you to awaken at 10:00 A.M.

"Ah, what a beautiful day!" you exclaim sarcastically from between your bed sheets. You might as well have been flattened by an eighteen-wheeler.

If you are reading this, you're probably one of the unfortunate souls who runs on zombie mode due to a lack of good Zzz's.

Take heart; you aren't alone. Many, if not most, Lyme disease sufferers wrestle with insomnia at some stage during illness. The causes of and solutions for sleeplessness are many. While not exhaustive, the following information is intended to provide insights and solutions to help jump-start your body back into sleep.

To begin with, liver toxicity is a big trigger for insomnia, especially if your body is trying to process loads of toxins. If you tend to awaken at 2:00 A.M. or not fall asleep until that time, this is a sign that your insomnia is related to the liver. Beware if you are hitting the Lyme critters hard and not doing enough detoxification protocol. To combat sleep deprivation related to liver toxicity, try one of the following remedies, which will help to mobilize toxins and carry them more quickly out of the body:

1. Chlorella. This must be from a pure source. Most commercial products are contaminated, so choose wisely. Mountain Rose Herbs, Premier Research Labs or E-lyte are good sources.

2. Coffee enemas. Yes, here it is again. Use only organic coffee and filtered water in a retention enema for ten minutes.

3. French green clay, zeolite and/or activated charcoal. As good sources of minerals, these products also mobilize toxins.

4. Liver detoxification supplements, especially milk thistle and herbal combination products such as Liv-52.

5. Glutathione. This amino acid complex mobilizes toxins and also helps the liver with phase two detoxification.

6. Epsom salt baths. These pull toxins from the body via the skin. Colder water produces better results.

Adrenal insufficiency is another cause of sleep deprivation. When the adrenal glands cannot synthesize the proper amount of hormones due to illness and stress, insomnia results. Supporting the adrenals in chronic illness is essential. J. Wilson, PhD, in his book, *Adrenal Fatigue, The 21st Century Syndrome,* offers some great suggestions for helping the adrenals. Personally, I have found that licorice, a high-quality Siberian ginseng such as that from HerbPharm and a low dose of pulsed natural cortisol, found in products like Isocort, have been effective for supporting my exhausted adrenals. Avoiding stress, sugar, caffeine and alcohol is likewise vital, as is maintaining a regular bedtime schedule. Having a small protein snack before bedtime will also help the adrenals to keep blood sugar levels stable during the night, which will prevent you from awakening.

Other endocrine abnormalities can contribute to insomnia. These include thyroid imbalance, pituitary dysfunction and hypothalamic suppression due to Lyme disease neurotoxins and other factors. Hypothyroidism can be treated with iodine or, if your body cannot synthesize thyroid hormone from iodine, synthetic or bioidentical thyroid hormone. Hyperthyroidism can also be treated with thyroid hormone, which serves to fix any imbalances and not necessarily increase thyroid hormone levels. Treating the pituitary gland and hypothalamus can be more difficult. If the problem is related to Lyme disease neurotoxins binding to these glands, then taking a toxin-binder such as mucuna bean powder or apple pectin can help to solve the problem. A few LLMD's administer growth hormone, HGH, which is normally produced by the pituitary gland, as a lack thereof has been implicated in sleep disorders.

Next, fixing any mineral deficiencies and ensuring an adequate intake of potassium, calcium and magnesium, especially at bedtime, will help to balance and relax the body. Having a snack containing the amino acid L-tryptophan is also beneficial. Cottage cheese, oatmeal and almonds are some good sources.

Pharmaceutical medications can be powerful for restoring sleep, but while most of them induce sleep, they tend to keep you from reaching delta brain wave sleep, which is crucial for restoration and repair of the body. Yet, they are good adjuncts when insomnia becomes severe, as they can help to "re-set" the body's clock. Trazodone is commonly prescribed, as are amitriptyline, lunesta, ambien and others. Mirtaza-pine is an anti-depressant that, in my opinion, could knock out an elephant, but carries side effects of weight gain and daytime drowsi-ness, at least temporarily. Sedatives such as lorazepam are also useful but are highly addictive and should only be used on a temporary basis.

Calming the mind and central nervous system through prayer, guided visualization or binaural beat CD's, (see: www.centerpointe.com), as well as performing other relaxation techniques, can also help you sleep, particularly if your disorder is related to anxiety or hyperactivi-ty. Herbal remedies are likewise calming, and chamomile, valerian, hops, Jamaican dogwood, lavender, rooibos and others are used in over-the-counter sleep formulas.

Every now and again, amino acids, such as GABA, 5-HTP and L-theanine, have proven to be helpful. Vickery (www.supernutrient.com) makes a good combination amino acid product. Amino acids and herbs did not work for me when I had severe insomnia, but Lyme disease sufferers have different needs, and if sleep problems can be mitigated by using a natural, rather than synthetic, product, this should always be the preferred form of treatment.

Finally, sleeping conditions matter! Go to bed and awaken at the same time every day. Make sure your room is dark and that you have all the necessary sleep gear to keep you slumbering, whether it be ear plugs, a face mask or a water pillow (to keep your neck from aching). Take a hot bath and have a snack before dozing off. Spend the last hour before bedtime doing something relaxing and if you can help it, don't fret about not sleeping. Consider that what you are going through will not last forever, painful as it may be right now.

<u>Fantastic Fixes for Low Energy</u>

Energy. We Lyme disease sufferers could all use a bit more of the stuff, and every little blip in our internal and external environments alters how much we have at any given moment.

Whether due to diet, climate, people, supplements, Jarisch-Herxheimer reactions or a symptom flare (to name just a few), it seems that Lyme disease sufferers are more vulnerable to reductions in energy than the average "healthy" human. We have less to begin with, so we must take precious care of what's given to us in order to maximize the rations. Following are a few suggestions for keeping the energy flowing.

Addressing thyroid and adrenal function should be a foremost consideration, since hormone levels dramatically affect energy. Perform a saliva cortisol and thyroid hormone test and treat the hypothalamus-pituitary-adrenal axis with herbs, vitamins and natural or synthetic hormonal supplements, as described in previous chap-ters. As much as possible, keep stress to a minimum, as this will help to balance your hormones.

Connie Strasheim

Then, examine your diet. I don't know about you, but certain foods down shift my body into putt-putt gear, especially those containing gluten and sugar. Other foods, such as dairy and eggs, are less of a problem for me, but they don't contribute to my energy bank, either. You'll have your own list of such foods. Pay attention to what time of day you have the least amount of energy and have some Popeye greens or other brightly colored veggies along with a protein your body can deal with, and save the fruit smoothie or oatmeal for a time when your energy is greater. It sounds obvious, but you'd be surprised at how many Lyme disease sufferers don't look closely at how food affects their energy, myself included. For two years, I ate almond butter with celery in the morning and justified the post-breakfast fatigue with the half-truth that nearly everything I put into my mouth in the morning leaves me exhausted. I have since found that switching to brown rice and turkey sausage has helped to mitigate the fatigue.

Next, spend time every day doing an activity you enjoy and with people around whom you can feel relaxed and happy. Emotions have a tremendous impact on energy levels, sometimes more so than physical or mental activities. Stay away from negative television programs, limit your time with critical or whiny people and fill your mind with uplifting thoughts. Funny movies can be good energy-boosters, provided they don't take your breath away because they make you laugh so hard!

Also, consider detoxifying your body on a regular basis. Keeping the organs working efficiently and the muck flowing outward with coffee enemas or toxin binders such as chlorella can provide you with an energy boost, as less garbage in the body means that everything functions better.

Supplements besides those that support the thyroid and adrenal glands can be helpful, but since the causes of fatigue in Lyme disease are multiple, it may be difficult to discern whether additional remedies will provide benefit. Nonetheless, other supplements that have proven to be helpful to Lyme disease sufferers include alpha-ketoglutaric acid, co-enzyme Q-10 and cordyceps mushroom.

Finally, get some rest! Stop trying to do so much when you are ill and turn off that computer at least an hour before bedtime, since computer light stimulates the pineal gland and disrupts the sleep/wake cycle.

Decreasing Your Symptoms by Increasing Serotonin

Lack of the neurotransmitter serotonin in chronic Lyme disease can do more than make you feel as though you've lost your personality. It exacerbates fatigue and pain, causes insomnia and makes a mess of your memory and cognition. The reasons for low serotonin range from not getting enough protein or fat, to adrenal fatigue, hypothyroidism and a lifestyle that isn't happiness-promoting. What's more, those darned Lyme critters are implicated in all of the above, as well as in other serotonin-depleting strategies.

Fortunately, serotonin levels can be increased in many ways, from medication to enjoying sunlight and activities that promote joy and well-being. They can also be raised through diet, which is what I focus here.

We always hear about turkey being high in tryptophan, an amino acid that is a precursor to serotonin. But who wants to eat turkey every day? While tryptophan sources aren't abundant, others besides turkey exist and are used by the body to make serotonin. Almonds, cottage cheese, oatmeal, peanut butter, shellfish, soy foods and tuna are some of these. If your digestion is poor, taking hydrochloric acid and digestive enzymes can aid in the body's uptake of these tryptophan-rich foods. If you are allergic to most, or all, of them, consider purchasing a 5-HTP supplement from the health food store, which is another precursor to serotonin, one step ahead of tryptophan in the amino acid chain.

Once tryptophan is inside the body, in order for it to become 5-HTP and then serotonin, the brain's biochemical pathways require that calcium and magnesium be present, as well as omega 3 and 6 fatty acids, B and C vitamins. Hormones are also involved, especially insulin and thyroid. Balancing the thyroid with iodine or supplemental

Connie Strasheim

thyroid hormone and getting enough insulin by eating plenty of complex carbohydrates will aid in the serotonin production assembly line, as will ensuring an adequate intake of vitamins and minerals.

Initially, some people may need more help than nutrients can provide and will have to resort to taking an anti-depressant medication. In the meantime, eating well and taking the above minerals, vitamins and fatty acids, along with other serotonin-enhancing strategies, can help to pull a sufferer out of the black pit of hormonal depletion, so that down the road, medication will no longer be necessary.

<u>Zoning in on the Ozone</u>

As already noted in previous sections, borrelia detests oxygen. It thrives in an anaerobic environment, which is one of the reasons why ozone therapy can be a superb adjunct to any Lyme disease protocol, because it increases tissue oxygenation by increasing elasticity and flexibility of red blood cells.

It also gives the immune system a boost to fight Lyme disease in other ways, by stimulating the production of white blood cells and tumor necrosis factor as it dramatically raises interferon levels. Tumor necrosis factor refers to a group of cytokines which are signaling compounds for inter-cellular communication and which play an important role in immune response. They are messengers that perform functions such as telling T-cells and macrophages where to go in the body to fight infection. Interferon is a protein naturally produced by the immune system in response to pathogens and which participates in a variety of inflammatory and immune reactions. Ozone likewise enhances the function of other immune agents, such as interleukin-2, one of the cornerstones of the immune system.

Ozone is beneficial for treating Lyme disease for other reasons. While it is not used as a primary bug killer for borrelia, it is yet anti-microbial and helps rid the body of opportunistic infections found in Lyme disease sufferers, including candida and mold.

Ozone accelerates the ATP cycle, which has the effect of increasing the body's energy and is great news for the chronically fatigued Lyme disease sufferer. It also makes the body's anti-oxidant enzyme system more efficient.

Indeed, the multiple benefits of ozone make it a useful adjunct in the treatment of Lyme disease. As previously mentioned, it can be taken via various methods, including rectal and ear insufflations, as well as saunas. Water and food can also be ozonated. For more information on ways to get your hands on some of this stellar stuff, including where to buy different kinds of ozone generators, check out: www.silvermedicine.org/ozonetherapy.html.

Avoiding Damaging Electromagnetic Fields

Did you know that your hair dryer and your clock radio could be hindering your healing from Lyme disease? Okay, so the damaging effects of these sources of electromagnetic fields on your body may be less significant than those of your cell phone or computer, but the burden that outside EMF's contribute to a body ridden with Lyme disease can be profound. Yeah, I know that your cell phone helps you to pass the time with a friend on your two-hour commute to work, and that the portable heater which warms your poor hypothyroid body in the winter feels so toasty. But consider that these, as well as any other device that you can plug into a socket, can affect your cells' energy and hinder your healing.

The damaging effects of EMF's seem to be a secondary concern for Lyme disease sufferers, as the harm done by these isn't quantifiable, and attention to other environmental toxins takes precedence, but if you believe that EMF's don't matter, then the following may change your mind.

Quantum Physics believes that all matter, including every cell in the body, is comprised of energy, and that inter and intra-cellular communication isn't carried out strictly on the level of biochemicals (that is, via hormones, cytokines and so forth) but also through energy channels in the body! In fact, some scientists believe that information transfer between energy signals is more efficient than through chemical signals (i.e., hormones).

According to Dr. B. Lipton, PhD, author of *The Biology of Belief*, external EMF's interrupt the body's energy signaling processes and cellular communication, with the result that DNA, RNA and protein synthesis and other cellular processes are disrupted. If we are really beings of energy as much as we are physical matter (or more so!) then why shouldn't our bodies be affected by electromagnetic frequencies?

Unless you live in a tent on an isolated beach in the Pacific (and even then you'd still get some EMF exposure), you can't completely avoid being affected by EMF's. It's not reasonable to assume that most of us can live as beach hippies on a remote corner of the planet, but we can reduce our exposure to harmful EMF's in a number of ways.

Minimizing cell phone use, unplugging appliances, (especially in the bedroom at night), purchasing a protective laptop screen, appliance diodes and EMF protection devices to wear on the body are a few ways you can safeguard your cells from damaging energies. One company that sells great EMF products is EnerCHIzer. These can be purchased online at: www.stairwaytohealth.com. Likewise, avoiding the frequent use of appliances such as hair dryers and fans, whenever possible, can help protect the body.

The Benefits of Sunshine

The sun gets a bad rap when it comes to Lyme disease. Proponents of the Marshall protocol believe that Vitamin D, from sunshine or supplements, can worsen Lyme disease symptoms, as Vitamin D is thought to help the L-form of the bacteria to proliferate. Lyme disease sufferers whose symptoms worsen in the sun or who have benefited from the Marshall protocol are likely to agree. Anyway, too much sun can weaken the immune system, and who needs that on top of an already beaten-down body? Studies have shown, however, that sunlight, when taken in small doses of just ten to twenty minutes a day, can be powerfully healing for Lyme disease sufferers.

Sunlight aids the immune system by increasing white blood cell counts and antibody levels and by stimulating neutrophils, a type of white blood cell, to engulf bacteria more rapidly. Also, many Lyme disease sufferers are loaded with toxins, and sunlight speeds the rate at which these get eliminated from the body. The Vitamin D produced from sunlight strengthens muscles and bones, while its rays stimulate the pineal gland to produce melatonin that is then converted into serotonin by day. Since these hormones work to correct mood and sleep disorders, this has positive implications for the depressed, insomniac Lyme disease sufferer. Further, sunlight makes trace minerals, which are important for a multitude of biochemical reactions, more accessible to the body. Finally, sunlight lowers cholesterol and triglyceride levels, as well as blood pressure and blood sugar, although these latter changes may be beneficial only for some people.

Like everything else in life, absorb a bit of this good thing in moderation. Doing so could have "sunny" effects upon your health.

The Perils of Tap Water and Finding A Suitable Water Filtration System

What's wrong with tap water? You may ask.

Nothing, if you don't mind a few heavy metals, toxic chemicals and pathogens entering your precious body. Tap water may be okay for folks with invincible immune systems, but, for the immune-compromised, its garbage may add a significant burden to a body struggling to overcome illness.

For starters, most Lyme disease and CFIDS sufferers have problems detoxifying heavy metals and other toxic chemicals found in water as a result of corroded pipes. Rumor has it that borrelia loves to sequester these metals, and plenty can be found in most commercial tap water systems. What's more, according to some sources, enforcement of safe chemical levels in water by the Environmental Protection Agency is inadequate.

Connie Strasheim

Flouride and chlorine are two other chemicals in tap water that are harmful to the body. Whoever decided that flouride was a great thing to put in toothpaste? Flouride and chlorine tear up DNA and cause neurological problems. Both have been associated with increased incidences of certain types of cancers and other diseases.

Finally, tap water is aswim with critters: parasites, bacteria and other organisms that wreak havoc upon the body. These persist despite the presence of chlorine, which is added to commercial water supplies, paradoxically, to kill the organisms. Again, a person with an amazing immune system can often contain or kill pathogens that enter the body via tap water, but the immune-compromised Lyme disease sufferer might not be so lucky.

Using a good, quality carbon block, reverse osmosis or, better yet, distilled water filtration system, can help to eliminate toxins in water. Distilled water is more beneficial to the body than water filtered by reverse osmosis or carbon block systems, as these remove decreasing levels of contaminants with each use. Such filters may become inefficient unless changed regularly, but they are less costly than a distilled water filtration system.

For a few hundred dollars, you can obtain an under-the-sink reverse osmosis or carbon block purifier. Multi-pure, www.multipure.com, is a good source. For a quality distilled water filtration system, check out Dolfyn, which may be obtained online at www.aquatechnology.net, as well as on other Internet sites. While a new system costs around $1,200, bargains can be often found on E-bay, www.ebay.com, for a quarter of the price.

Oh yeah, and just one more thing. Forget about bottled water. Its quality is also loosely regulated and much of it isn't any better than tap water. Besides, the plastic used to bottle water is toxic. If you must carry water around with you, you are better off using a glass or stainless steel bottle and filling it from home with your filtered water.

Chapter 6

Protocol Considerations

Distinguishing Herxes from Flare-ups and Relapses

Jarisch-Herxheimer, or pathogen die-off reactions, symptom flares and relapses mirror one another in their physical manifestations upon the body. They don't copy each other on purpose; it's just what happens in Lyme disease.

You have exceptionally bad brain fog one day and then a fever and chills on the next. On another day, your back aches something fierce, and fatigue waxes and wanes like the cycles of the moon. Lyme disease treatments, your diet, the moon and a half-dozen other sources of stress play a tug-of-war with your symptom picture besides.

So how in the wicked world of Lyme are you supposed to know whether your increased symptoms are a result of a flare caused by toxins, a relapse or a Jarisch-Herxheimer reaction?

Connie Strasheim

Good question. I'm still trying to figure that one out myself. You'd think that a few years of going through the Lyme disease die-off-improve-relapse rigamarole would have taught me a thing or two, but my body feels so random that at times I don't have a clue whether I'm moving backwards or forwards.

Herxing can produce an exacerbation of all Lyme disease symptoms, from fatigue to brain fog, to gut pain or whatever normally ails you, but life's stressors can do the same. A slip in the diet, the full moon or a fight with your spouse, and suddenly, you're swelling like a bloated cow on steroids.

Paying attention to when you are exposed to stress can enable you to discern flares from die-off reactions, although sometimes the effects of either aren't apparent. For instance, I can eat a piece of bread and the monster mood that the gluten produces won't rear its ugly head until the next day.

If my symptom exacerbation happens after a treatment, however, then I know I'm in herxheimer territory and not in the midst of a symptom flare, but discerning this can be a challenge, too, since some people herx immediately following a treatment, while others get the die-off reaction days later. Others don't seem to experience die-off symptoms at all.

So how do you know if a treatment is working and you are making progress if you aren't sure whether your increased symptoms are due to a herx, flare or, even worse, a relapse?

Perhaps the following will shed some sunlight (or moonlight!) upon the herx-flare-relapse dance.

1. Okay, so the bad news first. If you seldom experience herxheimer reactions and don't seem to be improving, not even a little over a period of many months, the protocol that you are doing probably isn't working. Further, if you have tried several different protocols with little to no improvement, consider that

borrelia may not be a primary player in your overall symptom picture.

2. If you seldom herx or can't discern herxes but still improve over a period of, say, six months or more, your protocol is working. You have superb detoxification mechanisms that allow your body to effectively remove Lyme toxins and thereby skirt the symptomatic effects of biotoxin removal.

3. If you experience a worsening of symptoms after a round of treatment, chances are, that treatment is effective for you. So keep going with your current protocol, no matter how many months it takes and even if you don't have major improvements. If you've been going at it for several months, however, you should start to notice minor changes. Beware of overdoing it. If the increase in symptoms feels continuous and relentless, then back down on your treatments or you may find yourself on a perpetual Jarisch-Herxheimer-merry-go-round with no getting off to discern progress.

4. If you have no idea which end is up, and your die-off reactions might as well be symptom flares, but you do feel okay sometimes, pay attention to whether the good days, sandwiched in-between the bad ones, are getting any better. Forget the bad days getting worse, as it isn't as reliable an indicator of progress as whether your good days are getting better.

5. If the bad days keep on getting worse, and the good days are becoming fewer, consider that the bugs might not be impressed with your ammunition, or that previously dormant infections have become active and are now taking the place of the old. Pathogens can be like the Russian doll factor. You remove a big one, only to find another, smaller one, inside. Or maybe you've been aiming at the wrong ones the whole time. Yet another possibility is that your body isn't effectively processing toxins, or you are relapsing due to environmental stressors or a protocol that's not suited to your needs.

Connie Strasheim

Don't despair; it may simply be time to switch therapies, focus on new strategies for removing toxins, or find out what new infection has cropped up so that you can treat it appropriately.

Finally, your healing can be hindered if you have congested detoxification pathways. Ensure that the liver, kidneys and other organs are in top working order by regularly performing detoxification protocol. This will enable treatments to work more effectively and help you to discern progress. Where there is congestion in the body, toxins cannot be released, and you will feel like a perpetual garbage dump, no matter how many anti-borrelia tactics you employ.

To Combine or Not to Combine Protocols, That Is the Question

Out of a desperate need to do anything and everything to heal, Lyme disease sufferers will often combine several Lyme disease protocols at once in order to throw as many weapons as possible at Borrelia and Company. In some ways, this makes sense. Since Lyme disease involves multiple infections and eradicating them is harder than trying to pull leeches from a leg, why shouldn't we do everything in our power to get rid of the suckers?

Unfortunately, when performed simultaneously, protocols can contradict one another, especially when they involve pharmaceutical or herbal antibiotics. I learned the hard way that spirochetes can hide from herbs, just as they can hide from pharmaceutical antibiotics. I notice that I can take an herb for about three to six months before I stop perceiving die-off reactions and improvement. When I remove the herb from my diet, the spirochetes that went dormant as a result once again became active, as evidenced by an immediate worsening of my symptoms and corresponding rise in my active infection load.

This isn't to say that pharmaceutical and herbal antibiotics don't have their uses, but if you decide to use them simultaneously with other protocols, such as Rife machines, salt/C or IRT, you may not receive the full benefit of one or more of these. Amongst the Lyme community at large, however, this theory remains speculative.

Below, I describe protocols that I feel can and cannot be effectively combined, based on my research and experience. For those that can be combined, please bear in mind that multiple, simultaneous therapies should be undertaken only when you are sure that you can tolerate the increased die-off reactions that will occur as a result. Also, you should be able to discern which therapies are working and which aren't, and this can be difficult if you are doing several at the same time.

1. The Salt/C protocol, Rifing, Quantum Techniques, Immune Response Training, The Healing Codes and other energy therapies may all be combined, because borrelia organisms cannot "hide" or develop resistance to any of these strategies, and energy-based therapies tend to work well with many different kinds of protocol. Salt/C and IRT are thought to be able to eradicate borrelia when it is in cystic form, though it may be more challenging or take longer than when the bacteria is in the bloodstream.

2. Immune Response Training and herbal or pharmaceutical antibiotics don't always work together well, in my experience. One particularly potent herb I used to take, andrographis, effectively chased my bugs into hiding so that IRT could not detect them. Once I stopped the herb, IRT was able to eradicate the bacteria. Many people start IRT treatments while taking antibiotics, which is fine at first, but you may encounter problems eradicating borrelia if you continue antibiotics for a prolonged period after commencing IRT sessions.

3. Rotating herbal and pharmaceutical antibiotics every few weeks or months may be more beneficial than doing just one type of therapy by itself, long term. This way, borrelia is always caught off guard and cannot develop resistance to any one particular drug or herb. By the way, nobody owns the monopoly on the "correct" antibiotic or herbal rotational schedule, as these mostly depend upon patient and practitioner experience. Also,

Rifing can be less effective if you are taking herbs or pharmaceutical antibiotics. However, pulsing Rifing with antibiotics, that is, doing one therapy for a time and then switching to the other, may render both strategies more effective.

4. Ozone and homeopathy can be used alongside many therapies, including IRT and antibiotics, and can enhance their effects.

5. MMS, Miracle Mineral Supplement, can be combined with many other treatments. It cannot be used with the salt/C protocol, unless doses of each are taken four hours apart.

Should You Pulse and Rotate Herbs, or Take Long-Term?

A tug-of-war exists when it comes to deciding upon a regimen for herbal antibiotics. On one end of the rope, are proponents for long, uninterrupted courses of herbs, while on the other, are patients and health care providers who advocate rotating short courses of different herbal remedies. Some favor both strategies, depending upon the infection and type of herb used, as well as patient reaction.

Consider that Borrelia and its cronies graduate at the top of the bacterial class when it comes to immune evasion and adaptability. They can change their camouflage, like a chameleon, and play hide-and-seek with whatever herbal or other antibiotic that is thrown at them. However, Borrelia and other infections don't like surprises, and short, unexpected courses of new herbal antibiotics are effective at throwing them off-guard so that they have no time to employ their tactics. Furthermore, when administered for short periods of time, Lyme disease sufferers are able to tolerate higher doses of herbs, which may render them more effective in the body. Pulsing can also be done for longer periods. For instance, I have found that taking andrographis continually for many months, with a week off every couple of months, has on occasion perpetuated a herxheimer reaction for me.

Past (and perhaps still current) protocols of Dr. Dietrich Klinghardt, M.D., Ph.D., have involved taking high doses of artemisinin for babesia, for approximately six days leading up to the full moon. Another LLMD, Dr. Lee Cowden, M.D., has advocated a twelve-day rotational protocol for borrelia and other infections using cumanda, quina and other herbs, with a three-day break taken in-between each one.

Proponents of long-term therapy generally don't believe that borrelia and other pathogens quickly develop resistance to herbs, and that long, uninterrupted courses are necessary in order for them to work well. S.H. Buhner, in his book, *Healing Lyme*, doesn't advocate pulsing anti-spirochetal herbs, including andrographis and cat's claw. He also doesn't advocate pulsing artemisinin for treatment of babesia as does Dr. Klinghardt. Buhner's and others' evidence for the effectiveness of long-term therapy may be just as valid as that found for those who pulse and rotate. This means that ultimately, each Lyme disease sufferer must go with his or her gut when formulating a plan, and discern his or her personal reactions to herbal treatments.

Whether or not you decide to pulse, if you can tolerate it, consider increasing your herbal doses around the full moon, as infections become more active then and great gains can be realized in getting the bugs when they are out and about. For a week leading up to the full moon, I used to take high doses of BioPure's ozonated rizol oils, which contain powerful bug killers such as walnut, clove, thyme, artemisia and garlic. I did not take them continuously, as the high doses, taken for many weeks, would have produced too many toxins for my body to eliminate. When used for just one week a month, however, they were quite effective.

I can't tell you which team to join in the tug-of-war. No right way to take herbal antibiotics exists. Many healthcare providers who administer herbs will agree that certain herbs work better when pulsed, and others when taken continuously for long periods of time. If you are unsure about whether to join the pulsing or long-term therapy team, do some research, find out how well others have fared on a particular protocol, and then pick a side and see how well you do.

Connie Strasheim

Getting the Most out of Herbal and Vitamin Supplements

We Lymie's sure spend a stash when it comes to treating our bodies with herbs and vitamins, don't we?

Sorting out which supplements a sufferer needs deserves an entire dissertation, which, lucky for you, I won't attempt to write today (or probably any other day!). What I will share are a few tips for making sure you get the most out of your supplements.

1. First, not all vitamins, minerals and herbs are created equal! Those you find at your local health food store may be good, but they may also have been sitting on the shelf for a long time, and therefore their potency is questionable. You might be better off ordering from a reputable company or asking your health food store for how long they allow supplements to sit on their shelves.

2. The elements of combination supplements may counteract one another, so choose wisely which ones you purchase. For instance, it is thought that calcium and magnesium use the same metabolic pathways in the body, so buying a product that contains both minerals may compromise its effectiveness.

3. Many companies use unhealthy fillers and preservatives in their products. If you see a fancy word you don't recognize on the ingredients label, watch out!

4. Supplements can come from contaminated sources. Consider fish oil. Unless the distillation process is impeccable, and the species of fish used is one that's less contaminated by mercury, you may receive a toxic product. It pays to do a bit of research on a product's harvesting, cultivation, storage and packaging methods.

5. Some products aren't manufactured in bio-available form, and the body cannot utilize what it can't break down or uptake. For instance, many people aren't able to metabolize vitamins in tablet form, because they have insufficient hydrochloric acid in their stomachs or not enough enzymes in the intestines to digest them.

6. Study the interactions between supplements, as their effects may cancel out one another. For instance, iron competes with magnesium for first place in the bloodstream, so these two minerals shouldn't be taken together. Vitamin C cancels out the effects of chlorella, and the list goes on. While you can't perceive and fix every possible interaction, a little knowledge can go a long way towards ensuring that you are getting the most from your products.

Why It's Good to Blast Critters on the Full Moon

Ever wonder why those werewolf and other grisly stories have been created around the full moon? Did you know that hospitals and prisons are busier during this phase of the lunar cycle as well? Guess what! The moon makes folks crazy and sick!

Yeah, I know the full moon is stunning and all, and if you think I'm party pooping all over this magnificent planet, I'm not. After all, it's not the moon's fault, but the organisms that live inside of us which cause the craziness.

Who knows why organisms come out to dance and copulate during the full moon, but one thing's for sure; if you are loaded with pathogens, you may feel terrible around the full moon as the bugs become more active in your body!

Most LLMD's recognize that Lyme disease symptoms tend to flare every four weeks. Some think that the flare coincides with a phase in borrelia's life cycle. I happen to think it's the full moon that does it.

Connie Strasheim

Personally, I'm annoyed that I often feel lethargic and moody during this lunar phase, but I've discovered that there is an advantage to the pathogens coming out to play; they become more susceptible to Lyme disease treatments! It isn't just the Lyme critters either, as other bugs get feisty during the full moon and are thought to be more susceptible to treatments, too.

So I nuke 'em hard during this phase. I double the dose of my herbal remedies for anywhere from three to six days prior to the full moon, or use my Rife machine on Full Moon Day. As a result, I'm often rewarded with a healthy dose of fatigue, brain fog or depression, and perhaps a colorful rash or cute little bartonella cat scratch, proof that I've indeed instigated an important die-off reaction.

Be careful, however! If you decide to ramp up on a treatment during the full moon, do so slowly and carefully, and with just one bug killer at a time until you know whether your body can tolerate the herxheimer reaction that is sure to follow. And if your symptoms are difficult enough to deal with as it is, then just take it easy on Full Moon Day. Declare it a holiday and rest, as you demonstrate compassion towards your friends and loved ones who are in a foul mood but don't seem to know why.

You Don't Need to Know about Every Little Infection in Your Body in Order to Heal

I used to think that if I could count all of my bugs, I would be alarmed at and in utter awe of how I'm able to function with such a party-fest of pathogens wreaking havoc on my biochemistry (or just napping away until the immune system gets knocked down again).

Fortunately (or unfortunately!) one day, I received insight into the "how many bugs" question when a friend tested me for a few thousand infections using a super high-tech device called a Harmonic Quad Zapper. The device found energetic frequencies in my body for roughly seventy-five different viruses, bacteria, parasites and other pathogens.

I probably have more. At the same time, I know that just because I carry the frequency for a particular pathogen, doesn't mean I have an active infection because of that pathogen. Some of the critters may be ghosts of past illnesses, others exist but live in a state of dormancy in my tissues, while yet others represent infections that are active and contributing to my current symptom picture.

I'll bet you have a bunch of bugs, too. Don't even bother trying to figure out what they all are and how to treat them. You'll drive yourself crazy, and besides, do you really want to know about every little organism living in your gut? If you have Lyme disease, take it for granted that you probably have one or more of the following active infections: candida, mold, fungus, babesia, bartonella, ehrlichia, rickettsia, Rocky Mountain spotted fever and mycoplasma.

In addition, in at least one of your two thousand blood draws over the past x-number of years, you probably tested positive for a herpes virus or two, Epstein-Barr, and a few other incidental bugs. Don't worry too much about these, at least initially; a high percentage of the population carries herpes, and ninety percent have high antibodies for Epstein-Barr. This doesn't mean that these viruses are currently causing you problems. Even if they are, they should probably be the least of your worries, because chances are, they can be brought under control once your Lyme disease and more virulent co-infections are treated.

Just don't get overwhelmed and think you have to get rid of all the bugs. You can't, and shouldn't, try to find a separate fix for all of them. So how do you know which ones to treat and which ones are active in your body?

Good question. To start, if you have a Rife machine, it might be beneficial to run frequencies for Lyme disease and the well-known major co-infections, including bartonella, babesia, ehrlichia and Rocky Mountain spotted fever, to see if you get a reaction. These all represent important infections that are likely to be contributing to your symptom picture and which therefore must be treated. Also, most Lyme disease sufferers have candida, mold and fungus issues to contend with, and treating these is also vital for recovery, so run the frequencies for those, too. You can also discover whether these infections are a problem for you by doing a trial run of an herb, pharmaceutical antibiotic or other treatment that is specific for each infection.

Next, taking a broad-spectrum anti-microbial such as colloidal silver or olive leaf and a good "catch-all" parasite cleanser such as Para 5 (prepared by Dr. R. Loyd of Health Balances in Seattle, Washington) will help eliminate many of the "biggie" infections, as well as mop up any miscellaneous ones.

For some of the minor infections, you can trust in your immune system's ability to "clean house" and mop them up, once borrelia and its major co-infections are under control. So before you start counting bugs, put together a broad-spectrum anti-pathogen protocol, along with one that is specific for borrelia and its major co-infections, as outlined above, and chances are, you'll eradicate a good portion of what's wreaking havoc upon your body. What infections you don't treat, you can deal with later, if, down the road, you still find that you have symptoms.

Trusting Your Gut when Making a Game Plan

With a plethora of available Lyme disease treatments and no one-shoe-fits-all protocol, how do you decide which ones to try?

Statistics on healing strategies and knowing what assortment of infections you're up against may get the wheels of decision moving. Although, inevitably, your unique biochemistry (along with Lyme specialists who disagree upon protocols) means that you'll have to come up with a way of sorting out every white lab coat's (or blue-collar's) professional opinion and come up with your own in order to discover which strategies best suit you.

Not being an expert in medicine, what do you do? Be an expert on your body instead and listen to your intuition! I believe this is one way in which God communicates to Creation, but even if you disagree with me, you've got to admit there's something awfully brilliant about that ol' gut feeling, isn't there?

You may not be accustomed to the quiet voice of intuition. You may find yourself ignoring it until you're in a life-or-death situation, in which case it tends to speak loudly, as in, "Quick! Get out of the building, because your attacker is coming to get you!" Yet, if you are still, if you move the busy thoughts and loud prejudices aside, you might hear its voice, telling you a thing or two about what your body needs. Listen to it and trust it, knowing that you've probably got too much wax in your ears to understand perfectly what it means to say, but that's okay. If you keep asking and listening and getting the same impression about a particular therapy, then perhaps that's the one to try next.

Before I knew I had Lyme disease, I instinctively felt that there was something wrong with my adrenal glands, and I had this vague feeling from day one that I needed to pay serious attention to them, whatever illness ailed me. Even though I now know that I have Lyme disease, the belief that I also suffer from severe adrenal fatigue has been solidified through lab test results and correlating symptoms. It isn't my whole problem, but my gut has wisely been whispering admonitions left and right that I support my endocrine system in order to heal from Lyme disease.

When formulating a healing plan from amongst a multitude of treatment options, stop, open your ears and keep listening as you go about your day. Trust that feeling which pokes at you from deep within, that feeling you're not sure about but which hangs around nonetheless. It may be trying to tell you something important about which road to take when the light turns green and it's time to go.

Getting Rid of the Inner Quack and Learning to Trust Alternative Medicine

In the western world, our minds have been soaped n' scrubbed into believing that unless a healing remedy and its results can be measured, quantified and substantiated by a blood, urine, sweat or other bodily fluid test, then that remedy is useless. We have been taught to close our minds to the methodologies of the eastern world, which rely upon therapies whose results cannot be substantiated except by unconventional testing methods and testimonials of patients. In the western world, these methods are labeled as "alternative," as though they should be back-ups to the trusty pharmaceutical drugs we've come to rely upon here.

Granted, some Lyme sufferers are wary of "alternative" medicine, because they have been wounded by outside-the-box therapies that did not deliver what they promised, and have encountered quacks with big orange feet and snakes that have swindled thousands of dollars from their wallets. Then there are those who just don't want to give up the comfy old shoes of pharmaceutical medicine.

But what if the inter-workings of an effective remedy cannot be explained by what we know in the western world? What if we have been given the What without the How or the Why? Should we conclude that the remedy doesn't work?

It's as if we expect every solution to every health malady that ever existed to fit within the parameters of our limited and biased testing devices, when sometimes, the only proof that a remedy works is found in healed flesh and bone.

Just because you can't understand a protocol, doesn't mean it isn't worthy. Just because it isn't well-known. Just because it seems about as plausible as purple cows sprinting over the moon. Just because its testing methods rely upon undefined science. If others have been healed by it, or if in your gut you believe it could work, then why shouldn't you try it?

Doing so doesn't necessarily require more faith than taking a tested-and-only-sometimes-true pharmaceutical antibiotic. After all, these have failed to heal many Lyme patients (just as alternative methods have). Yet, isn't it funny how alternative methods tend to suffer a heavier societal beating when they don't deliver what they promise?

Sometimes, treading an unconventional healing path means becoming the black sheep and taking a leap into yonder, away from the safe pastures that others know, because your gut or your god or your healed neighbor are telling you to go.

To those who are afraid of finding Dr. Quack behind every alternative therapy, I encourage you to throw the old comfy shoes away. To dare to be the black sheep, to take the less-trodden road and, if you believe in God, to turn to the Great Physician and ask for discernment. Real solutions are often found off the beaten path.

Connie Strasheim

Chapter 7

Heavy Metals

The Importance of Ridding the Body of Heavy Metals and Choosing a Chelation Method

It's no secret that heavy metal toxicity is becoming a big problem worldwide. The high prevalence of mental disorders is thought to be due in part to toxicity from mercury, lead, aluminum and other metals—especially mercury, which is significantly more toxic than lead or aluminum.

While we can't completely control the amount of metal that enters our bodies, doing things such as drinking purified water, eating organic food, especially wild fish (instead of farm-raised) and not getting dental amalgams(or having them removed by a metal-literate dentist, which is crucial), can help keep body levels down.

Being infected with Lyme disease presents a special problem when it comes to heavy metal toxicity, as Borrelia and Company are thought to sequester metals. When the bugs die, they release these metals into the body; hence, a person who tries to fix their metal problem before treating Lyme disease may make incomplete progress. Add to this the

Connie Strasheim

fact that metal chelation can take years. Further, Lyme disease sufferers tend to have detoxification problems and are likely to accumulate and retain metals at a greater rate than a person with fewer health problems.

Metal chelation is an art unto itself, which, if done improperly, can re-distribute metals into the body, causing more problems than if the metals had just been left alone. Much controversy exists over what constitutes a safe, effective chelation method.

Chlorella and cilantro are widely used by many, but these agents are thought to form imperfect bonds with mercury, allowing for the possibility of its re-distribution into cells if it's dropped by the chelator on the way out of the body. Chlorella, if it is of good quality, is generally thought to be safe and effective, but these factors are also influenced by a person's biochemistry.

Some good chlorella products to try are those made by Biopure, E-lyte and Premier Research Labs. The variety C. pyreneidosa is thought to absorb toxins best, though some people have trouble digesting it and prefer other types.

Cilantro mobilizes more toxins than it can carry out of the body, but some believe it to be safe if chlorella is simultaneously taken to mop up the excess toxins. Also, cilantro is often heavily contaminated, but by adding cilantro leaves or tincture to hot tea, these toxins can be removed. Dr. Klinghardt, M.D., believes cilantro to be the only chelation agent capable of mobilizing mercury stored in the intracellu-lar space; that is, that which is attached to structures such as mitochondria, liposomes, and so forth, and is therefore an important adjunct to chlorella.

Other heavy metal chelation experts, such as A. Cutler, PhD, would say that taking chlorella and cilantro to rid the body of heavy metals is risky. He contends that DMSA or DMPS with alpha-lipoic acid are more appropriate methods, as these agents form stronger bonds with metals and are therefore safer. The drawback to DMSA is that it must be taken on a regular schedule, every four hours or so, even during the night. It can also produce side effects, as can DMPS.

Finally, PCA-Rx by Maxam Labs is a spray that removes heavy metals through a process called clathration, whereby the toxin is completely encapsulated by the chelating agent, thereby preventing it from being dropped on the way out of the body. It also has virtually no side effects. For this reason, it's thought to be safe as well as quite effective. The only drawback to this product is its price, which may cost up to $125 a month. This is about twice the cost of a protocol involving chlorella and cilantro.

Other chelation methods exist, such as glutathione and zeolite products such as Natural Cellular Defense, but those listed above are the most commonly used at present.

When formulating a detoxification plan, the cost of therapy is an important factor to consider, since heavy metal chelation often needs to be performed for many months, if not years. While chlorella and cilantro may be riskier agents, they may be the only option if you are on a tight budget. Taking small doses to start off with can help determine how you will react to them. Or, if you can afford it, try PCA-Rx, or perhaps the Cutler protocol.

Removing heavy metals from the body accelerates healing from Lyme disease. Indeed, some people may not experience total health until this aspect of illness is addressed.

The Power of Minerals to Remove Metals

Heavy metals are thieves. They steal the receptor sites on cells normally reserved for minerals. Wherever the body is deficient in minerals, receptor sites hold up Vacancy signs, and heavy metals move right in. Once there, the metals become a nuisance to get rid of.

As Lyme disease sufferers, our bodies are hit with a triple whammy. As previously mentioned, a weakened immune system means that we can't chelate heavy metals out of the body as effectively as a healthier person can, and it is rumored that borrelia is keen on sequestering metals for its survival. The bacteria also gobble up our mineral reserves and mess with our metabolism so that nutrients don't reach the cells, which means that more mineral receptor sites are left wide open for metals to attach to.

How do we remedy this? Besides undertaking an aggressive chelation protocol, we need to chug minerals, minerals and more minerals! And not just the macrominerals, such as magnesium and potassium, but the seventy or so trace minerals found in our bodies. This can be accomplished with regular dosing, that is, two or more times a day, of the macros plus a good quality trace mineral complex product, such as Concentrace. As Lyme disease sufferers, we may require doses larger than those recommended on bottles. I use my intuition and muscle-testing when deciding upon how much to take, but you may want to get a good hair analysis test to help you determine your level of deficiency, keeping in mind that this testing procedure also has its limitations.

Keeping an adequate supply of minerals in the body not only ensures that the immune system will have the resources it needs to function and fight Lyme disease, but also discourages and displaces heavy metals from binding to sites that are rightfully reserved for these precious minerals.

Section II

Lifestyle Strategies for Healing Lyme Disease

Connie Strasheim

Chapter 8

Diet and Supplements

Self-discipline in Your Diet

"If I have to do this diet another day, I'm gonna...."

Wait! Don't jump! It's not worth it. Honestly, this will all be over one day. Just think of those starving kids in Africa. Seriously. Have a look through a World Vision magazine and try to appreciate what's on your plate. So you can only eat two green vegetables and a bit of wild salmon. At least you get to eat every day.

But I sympathize with what you are going through. I, too, turn into a jealous toad in the presence of a friend who is gobbling away at her lemon pie. At the same time, I know that my health is worth the sacrifice.

Oh yeah? You say.

I know. It sucks. Despite your efforts to avoid the truffles and red wine and every condiment under the sun and despite the fact that you've eliminated all grains, dairy, legumes and fruit from your diet, you still relapse. All that struggle and discipline seems to be for nothing. Your

Connie Strasheim

reward is more fatigue, more pain, and you might as well eat a candy bar the size of a rhino.

And, yes, if you have to endure another day of this, you're going to crack like an egg dropped from a ten-story building. I've walked along that ledge, too...and I confess, I've jumped. Many times.

And whenever I break against the pavement, I shout, "Woo hoo! The diet's over and so is the battle against Lyme disease (temporarily, anyway). But who cares, bring out the champagne, strawberries and chocolate, because man, it's been too long and I really don't give a flying fungus whether I eat wild salmon or whipped potatoes! Speaking of fungus, the one in my liver is going to expand into all of my guts after I finish these au gratin potatoes. And maybe Borrelia will have some champagne with me and reproduce like a bacteria on steroids, but heck, at least I don't have to deprive myself any longer of this yummy stuff!"

Okay, so who am I to tell you to hang in there, that the stringent diet's worth it?

Maybe you do have to cheat occasionally and suffer a setback.

On the other hand, if you're able to remember those kids in Africa or just be grateful for being able to eat two foods, knowing you will reap the benefits of health down the road, then you might want to think twice about that lemon pie or high-glycemic carrot.

From personal experience, I know that one little cheat erases entire energy treatments for me and renders other therapies less effective. Further, muscle testing indicates that my infections have a multiplication-fest at the mere introduction of a marshmallow into my body.

Don't tell me. What about Lola Lymefree who ate whatever the dickens she liked and went into remission? Sorry guys, I think the Lola's of the Lyme world are few. Go ahead, disagree with me. I don't own anyone's truth but my own, and even mine is subject to revision.

Just don't jump off the diet. Tell yourself you'll do it for a day, then a week, then a month, and then pay attention to your symptoms. Perhaps you'll notice changes that will make the effort worth it. Persevere, or pray for another way that won't make you crazy. Or, if you must be liberated from the tedium of discipline, jump, and then allow the cheat to strengthen your resolve.

Avoiding Harmful Food Additives by Learning the Language of Deception

If you want to keep your brain and body functioning as you recover from Lyme disease, you're going to have to learn a new language besides English in order to read the ingredients on food labels. That new language is called Deception, and it will help you to identify the neurotoxic additives on food labels that cannot be spotted by plain English alone. Companies are getting smart and are learning to cloak poison in sweet-sounding verbiage, so that you're fooled by the actual content of what's in your food and supplements. So I'm here to give you your first lesson in the language of Deception, so that you can better identify these toxic additives.

Since MSG, monosodium glutamate, is troublesome for many, let's start here. MSG falls into a class of neurotoxins called excitotoxins, which cause seizures, abnormal nerve development, neuron destruction, learning problems and migraines. They are implicated in a myriad of neuropsychiatric and neurodegenerative disorders, including Parkinson's, Alzheimer's and ALS.

In the language of Deception, MSG may be called any one of the following:

Hydrolyzed vegetable protein
Vegetable protein
Textured protein
Hydrolyzed plant protein
Soy protein extract
Caseinate

Connie Strasheim

Yeast extract
Natural flavoring

Yup, you heard right. Natural flavoring. I couldn't have come up with a better translation in the language of Deception myself. We all want what's natural, since natural things are good for the body, right? Sorry, but I don't think there is any way to describe MSG as a natural ingredient in vegetables or any other healthy food.

Don't think that MSG is the only excitotoxin out there, either. At least seventy-five others have been identified. You will find these in almost all processed foods, so the best way to avoid these toxins, besides learning the language of Deception, is to steer clear of such products.

In the meantime, you might want to find out if someone has compiled an English-Deception dictionary, because eight translations for MSG are an awful lot to memorize. Besides, an additional twenty-eight hundred substances are used as food additives, and you never know how many of these are harmful and disguised on food labels in the language of Deception.

So Many Lyme Diets, So Much Confusion: Choosing a Regimen that Works

The number of so-called healthy diet plans out there could fill a few thousand libraries. As Lyme disease sufferers, we can narrow our focus to a half-dozen, as food allergies preclude others from possibility. Still, doesn't it seem that the more you know about nutrition, the more questions you ask yourself about which diet to pursue?

Some of the questions you may ask yourself are: Do I cut out fruit? After all, fruit can cause a blood-sugar spike and supposedly feeds the Lyme bacteria. Do I eliminate grains, including brown rice, because they might exacerbate my leaky gut and cause inflammation? Do I exclude red meat or chicken because these are acidic to the body? Do I skip fish because it's loaded with mercury? What about dairy? Is cow's milk really all that bad for you? Should I forego anything that's not organic because it's loaded with toxins and void of nutrients? Do I follow the Ayurveda, Blood Type, South Beach, or Maker's diet? What about a combination of the above?

Most health-conscious Lyme disease sufferers and nutritionists would probably agree upon only one thing when it comes to diet: organic green vegetables are good for you! The rest of what we call food is up for debate, as you can find a good reason (allergies being the foremost) not to eat from any of the other food groups, but you must eat something besides greens!

So beyond food sensitivities and allergies, how do you decide, amongst conflicting opinions, what to eat? Below find my suggestions, which have less to do with the inherent nutrients in food and more about your body's response to them.

Start by considering how a particular item makes you feel shortly after you ingest it. If you get droopy-eyed and feel like a slug, it's probably a no-go.

Secondly, with what ease can you digest it? Does it take you a 90-minute flick to finish a raw spinach salad? Does it come out the other end looking the same as when you put it into your mouth? These are signs that it's time to either sauté the item or choose a different food.

Third, amongst your selections, are you able to marry decent amounts of fat, protein and carbohydrate at every meal? If not, it's time to find a partner or two for that carbohydrate.

Fourth, do your meals keep your belly happy for longer than an hour? Aim for enough protein-carbohydrate-fat to keep the motor going for at least a few hours.

Fifth, have you learned to detest mealtimes because you can't stand broccoli and salmon but feel you should eat them anyway? Find healthy alternatives from the garden and the sea.

Connie Strasheim

Sixth, are you gaining or losing weight on your diet? If you are noticeably under or overweight, re-evaluate your plan.

Seventh, is it important to your emotional well-being to eat foods high in sugar? If so, have a slice of chocolate cake every now and again without going wild.

Finally, and most importantly, learn to muscle test yourself for foods (as discussed previously). This is an applied kinesiology technique that reveals *exactly* what your body wants from each of the five food groups. Your results from this test may surprise you, as you will find that you are able to eat some foods that are shunned in popular Lyme circles, and vice versa.

Becoming Liberated from Pill Fatigue by Eliminating Unnecessary Supplements from Your Diet

Which supplements and medications should you take? Isn't that the eternal Lyme disease question? So many factors to consider. Money. Bugs. Which busted up parts of the body could use a bit more help.

You're ten years into your healing journey and still wondering about the positive effects of the pharmacy in your kitchen, bedroom and bathroom. You've spent thousands, stressed over pill-popping schedules and become the champion of vitamin-supplement gobbling. You're ready to declare Pill Fatigue.

Surely some of this stuff has kept you functional, perhaps even alive, but separating the products that have contributed to your wellness from those that have been sent straight to the other end of the digestive tract has been difficult to discern, hasn't it?

Consider first your vitamins and minerals. Maybe you should give up on fixing the lack of every little vitamin B-this and B-that, even though your physician told you that you are deficient in most of the B-vitamins. Some nutritionists would say that trying to fix one nutritional imbalance creates others. It's like a game where none of the pieces ever fit together properly. Give the body a little zinc and the next thing you know, it needs iron, too. Maybe it would be better to just take a multi-vitamin. While the same problem exists with taking a blanket supplement, perhaps it's less risky than taking mega-doses of a single nutrient. Plus you'll save a few dollars. Keep your fish oil, magnesium and a bottle of trace minerals, too, as their benefit is nearly indisputable for Lyme disease sufferers. Magnesium might be the only single supplemental mineral that's recommended for all Lyme disease sufferers, since borrelia gobbles up the stuff like candy.

Now, take a look at your bug killers. It's good to pick a protocol and stick with it for awhile, but when you get that nagging feeling like your spirochete friends are getting used to your herbal or antibiotic regimen, it's time to put those herbs or drugs aside, at least temporarily. Also, when you have fewer supplements to juggle, it will be easier to discern which ones are helping you.

Next, consider the other crutches that you think you need for proper biochemical function, such as hormones, immune system boosters and anti-coagulants. Yes, this is challenging, as not having enough thyroid hormone can be a BIG deal. If you are taking a low dose, however, you might try tapering it off to see if your body can deal with the change.

As you ponder which supplements to toss, consider whether the evidence of their effects upon your body is measurable and concrete. Maybe it's not the thyroid hormone that you need to get rid of. Maybe it's the transfer factor, whose effects upon your body are dubious or unknown. If you're not sure, take it on a vacation to the pantry or to a friend's house and see if your body, in its soul of souls, can live without it.

Round off your downsizing project by having a second look at your detoxification agents. I used to take chlorella, cilantro and French green clay, in addition to a liver and kidney cleansing herbal combination. Now I wonder why in the blessed name of borrelia I needed all of these. One key detoxification product, chlorella, might have been

Connie Strasheim

sufficient, and I could have supported my liver and kidneys with a proper vegetable diet.

If you feel toxic as a trash heap, however, don't necessarily follow my lead. Your body may need more than one garbage remover, since detoxification supplements vary in their uses. For example, chlorella removes mercury from the gut, but not the brain. If mercury is a problem for you, you'll want to add cilantro to your chlorella, or try a different product altogether. Just be aware that the liver has to detoxify everything that enters your body, and if you take too many supplements, these can actually be a burden, not a blessing, to your health. In the end, it's not just about the pocketbook or the tedium of taking pills, but also your body's ability to handle these, too.

Now, isn't it liberating to be free of so many gelatin capsules? Go ahead; see how enthusiastically your body responds to the decision to be free of pill fatigue. I wish you blessings upon your pocketbook in the meantime!

The Benefits of Maté

No, I don't mean mate as in your spouse or, as the term is used in Australia, your buddy!

I'm referring to maté (pronounced mah-tay), a South American tea that's extraordinarily rich in nutrients. This tea is thought to have more antioxidants than white, black or green tea and is loaded with magnesium and potassium, minerals that are deficient in most Lyme disease sufferers. When drunk from a gourd (or "calabaza") and a closed-ended metal straw with holes, as is the custom in South America, the tea is exceptionally potent and satisfying.

When I lived as an exchange student in Argentina I didn't care much for it, and frankly, I didn't understand the Argentine culture's fascination with it. Ten years later, however, with Lyme disease symptoms striking me full-fledged, I discovered huge bags of this tea at a Mexican supermarket in Denver and tried it again, this time falling passionately in love with it for the powerful effects that it had upon my body.

How could it be that I hadn't noticed the amazing benefits of maté before? Within a half-hour of consuming the beverage, my body aches and brain fog would dissipate, as my energy increased and spirits lifted. Truly, this tea was akin to a drug for me.

For nearly a year, I craved the stuff like crazy, and I believe it supplied my body with much-needed nutrients. It has also been known to stimulate detoxification reactions in some Lyme disease sufferers, which suggests that it may also have been useful to me as a detoxifying agent.

I would still be drinking it every day were it not for its caffeine content, which is hard on the adrenal glands. Yes, maté can be as bad as coffee in this regard, especially when taken South American style. However, if drunk in moderation, the tea can be a tremendous benefit to the body, especially for those with relatively healthy adrenal glands.

Connie Strasheim

Chapter 9

Exercise

Choosing an Exercise Plan that Will Get You Moving but Won't Leave You Wiped Out

For a year following my crash from Lyme disease, I was in denial about my body's capacity to handle exercise. To prove to myself that I wasn't that bad off, and at least once or twice a month, I'd valiantly join friends on two-hour long hikes or partake of intense hour-long skating sessions in the park. Such activities would leave me wasted for a day or two afterwards, but it took me awhile to wise up and realize that this kind of exercise wasn't beneficial for me. After I stopped fooling myself and switched to gentler workouts, my body responded by rewarding me with greater stamina, instead of exhaustion, after my sessions.

As Lyme disease sufferers, we must keep our limbs moving, and that means more than just making it to the toilet and the kitchen every day, but it doesn't mean killing ourselves in the name of health, either. Following is what I've learned about formulating a fitness regimen through my trials-and-errors of exercise.

Connie Strasheim

First, knowing what exercises to perform and how much when you are ailing can be like fine-tuning a piano. A little too much of this, not enough of that, and the body suffers or doesn't get what it needs. You must learn what types of exercise will make your cells sing with rejuvenation and not sputter with exhaustion. It might mean a light yoga session, or a walk out in the sun, or an easygoing swim at the gym. It is generally agreed that most Lyme disease sufferers should not perform any kind of high-impact aerobic activity, as this stresses the heart and burns out the adrenal glands. Some LLMD's, such as J. Burrascano, believe that stretches and weight training using small weights are important for Lyme disease sufferers, so you may want to alternate these with a low-intensity aerobic activity such as walking. Even if you're really sick, try making a few laps around the house in your Winnie-the-Poo jammies, with two-pound weights strapped to your ankles.

After you decide upon a beneficial form of exercise, you must then consider the intensity and frequency of your workout. Maybe you can manage a day-long bike ride without collapsing on your face, but how much of a beating is your body supposed to take in the meantime? With one workout, have you pushed yourself to the point of now needing a nap for the next three days?

Conversely, if the thought of a shiny forehead or moving those legs two feet out the front door leaves you terrified you'll break like blown glass, consider that by using your fragility to rationalize your inactivity, you'll keep your bugs happy by your anaerobic activity. Borrelia adores that you aren't feeding it oxygen! Even if you really, truly cannot make it to the mailbox, start by opening that front door and stepping outside. Make it your goal to get to the driveway within a week, and then to the mailbox in another. Or if you are bedridden, try some leg lifts or arm raises. Just move your limbs however you can.

Finally, working out every other day, for a half-hour to an hour, seems to be the optimal frequency for most Lyme disease sufferers. A day of rest in-between will enable you to shake the mild post-exertional fatigue that may follow your workout.

Chapter 10

Relationships

"I'm too Sick to Be in a Romantic Relationship" ... Or Are You, Really?

Is this just another one of your excuses for staying single? Or is it an idea based on your friends' marriages, struggling because one of the partners has Lyme disease? Or is it a conclusion you've drawn as a result of your own negative experiences of having dated while sick? While being in a relationship can be challenging and impractical when you are multi-symptomatic, how about we hash it out right here and re-think whether there's any chance that romantic relationships are possible with this illness?

Let's start with dating. Since I'm writing from a woman's perspective, I'm going to present a scenario in which the protagonist is female. No offense, guys, but last time I looked, I didn't have chest hair so I can't effectively understand your unique challenges as men with Lyme disease. Society expects you to be providers, and in some ways, I think your dating and relationship issues are more difficult than what we women face, but I think you'll be able to relate to the following, anyhow.

Connie Strasheim

We live in an activity-based society, and if you are a woman with Lyme disease and can't participate due to physical or mental limitations, you might think you aren't worth the effort for most guys. Sure, you could find yourself a dude who doesn't need stimuli galore, but even if you managed that, would he travel to your house in the boonies and pay for your recreation (since you're broke) every time you happen to feel well enough to go out? Anyway, what John Dopey-eyes wants to spend half his nights on the sofa, just hanging out? Especially when he could date cute Christie the cyclist, who is cool and collected and...absolutely active. Why would he trade this for a night on the sofa with you, the Loony-Tunes Lymie? Absolutely what benefit would he derive from dating a motionless, mopey woman?

Okay, so you're not manic or bedridden, but Lyme disease does bring on some frigid seasons fraught with fear, rage and fatigue, and during those times, you're not even useful to yourself, never mind exciting company for a boyfriend.

What's more, you can't often laugh because it steals the wind from you, you can't be witty and articulate because of brain fog, and you can't go dancing because you have postural hypotension. You can't eat at the coolest Italian restaurant in town because pasta makes you swell like a hippo with hives, and you can't stay out late because you need ten hours of sleep. You often cry and beat your bed pillows because you're bone tired, and you're anxious and irritable because your brain is loaded with pathogens. Yeah, you reckon you're about as much fun as a pole in the ground.

Then there's the commitment thing. What if you ended up canceling half your dates because of unpredictable fatigue? Would your beau be able to smile and say, "Hey, no problem!" What if all of your exciting Saturday night engagements ended at 9:00 PM?

And supposing John Dopey-eyes did make it past the sofa spud dating stage, would he be keen on financially supporting a woman who couldn't work because of her illness? Would he hang around if he discovered that Lyme disease is a contender in the race for the world's next worst sexually transmitted disease (STD)? You decide that such a soul would have to be possessed by God to want to endure the possibility of such hardship. And this is just the beginning! What if you actually got married?

On the other hand, maybe this scenario is just a replacement for your previous excuses for not dating. The old broken record that sings, "You're not good enough for any man because..." (and then fill in the blank). Consider that there will always be a blank if you want one to be there.

Anyway, didn't God create human beings to give and receive love? Should illness preclude you from enjoying the benefits of dating or being loved by another? Don't Lyme disease sufferers need to love others, as well as be loved in return? Should you put your life on hold until you can make yourself more perfect for Mr. or Mrs. Right? Isn't love more dependent upon the eye of the beholder than the qualities of the beloved? Not that you don't have any positive qualities just because you are sick!

But do your handicaps make you less loveable? Why are you focusing on the minuses, anyway? Even if they were minuses, isn't everyone physically or mentally handicapped somehow?

You concede that the benefit of finding a man in your condition is that you'll quickly weed out the superficial ones. Those who need recreation in order to have joy in a relationship. Those who can't handle a few tears or who want Wonder Woman instead of the mortal human. And those who don't have enough compassion to see who you are, beyond your illness. All these guys get pushed to the wayside as soon as they learn about your infirmity. It saves a lot of wasted time and energy, doesn't it? (However, be forewarned, there will be some who will nonetheless think that they can handle your illness and will insist that things will work out fine, but it's only because you look and act so darned healthy!).

So what do you have to offer?

Connie Strasheim

Your mind wanders to the lessons you've learned, and are still learning, as a result of your ten-year journey with Lyme disease. These lessons seem to be greater than those that were given to you during the first forty years of your life.

To start, you're learning to value yourself for who God has made you to be, instead of for your accomplishments. Boy, hasn't that been a tough one for the skull! You're learning to cherish and nurture yourself, because if you don't, you know that you'll be in this Lyme fix forever. You know what it means to take care of yourself and to set healthy boundaries with others, for the sake of your sanity as well as theirs.

You now have more compassion towards others. Knowing that a glowing complexion and bright eyes are often found in the sickest of people, you no longer frown at the handsome young man in the grocery store who pays for his goods with food stamps, or your so-called lazy cousin who can't seem to hold down a job.

You don't judge your neighbor who has fits of rage over the garbage cans you leave outside, because you know what it means to live with mental dysfunction.

You no longer become irritated at friends for not remembering your birthday, because you know what it's like to have a memory like a flea and having expectations of others only depresses you and is detrimental to your health.

You don't resent friends and family for not understanding your pain, because you don't know what they have suffered, either. Besides, bitterness over what others cannot do or be for you is toxic to your body, and for your own sake, you'll have none of it. So you no longer try to change others because you know you can only change yourself. You may still fly off the handle at times, but you are aware of your dysfunction and are working tirelessly to become whole again, because now the stakes are higher.

You have come to appreciate the kindness of others who have helped you through your trials, which leaves you hoping you can do the same for another someday.

You have drawn closer to God because there's no way you could have made it through this illness without Him. In moments of forced solitude and desperation, you have heard His voice and know that He has been teaching you how to love yourself and others more deeply so that you can be fully healed, from the inside out.

Haven't these lessons fostered in you some fine qualities to offer another?

No, you really don't have much to give John Dopey in terms of recreational companionship, but you do have much to offer in depth of character, and that doesn't even include that spectacular character you had before you got sick! You've always been able to listen to others, to offer sage advice, and are reasonably good company, most of the time. You haven't changed; you just have more off-days. At the same time, the lessons that Lyme disease has taught you mean that you might be more healed than before you even knew you were sick! Anyway, if John Dopey's character is anything like yours, he'll be willing to handle your off-days, however frequent they may be. For love is patient and kind, and seeks not its own.

Yeah, maybe relationships, if they are based on recreation and lots of externals, just aren't worth it for Lyme disease sufferers. When it comes to developing a more meaningful connection, however, then even you, the world's most disabled Lyme disease sufferer, can participate!

They Will Never, Ever Understand: Learning to Accept Your Family's and Friends' Emotional Limitations

They won't understand. No matter how hard you try to explain the suffering that Lyme disease causes you and how much they attempt to empathize with your pain. Unless they have Lyme disease, too, they won't get it. With your help, they may grasp certain aspects of your suffering better, but they'll never be able to jump inside your skin and know what you are going through, and frankly, many won't want to. Their problems keep them occupied and having to empathize with you or support you in any way may be asking too much.

Don't bother talking yourself blue in the face, trying to justify to them why you can't work. Why you can walk a mile but can't go shopping. Why you need organic food at every meal, and why loud places, people and perfume are a big deal. Your loved ones have never seen an ill person look so darned healthy, and your behavior contradicts what a sick person is supposed to act like. Their idea of illness is a person with cancer, not you. It's someone who is pale, has dark circles under his eyes and who can barely move. While that may describe you, you've also been known to go dancing from time to time, and how is it possible for a person to be sick and swing dance?

Even more baffling is your social behavior. Telling your family that Lyme disease has affected your memory won't stop them from wondering why you can't remember to turn off the stove and why you seem to pay no attention to the little details that they share with you about their lives. Your bouts of unexplained sadness will be a mystery to them. While they know it's no fun to be sick, they will yet wonder why you can't just pull yourself up by your bootstraps and be a little happier. They won't comprehend why you always leave social gatherings early and why you can't listen to their detailed, drawn-out stories as often as they'd like.

Not only will your family and friends not understand your symptoms and social problems, they also won't grasp the financial hardship you endure because of Lyme disease. Those whom you expect to give you a few hundred bucks to help pay your rent won't offer you a dime, and those whom you don't expect to help you, just might do so. Also, your friends' and family's idea of hardship may be having no money in a retirement account, while yours is not being able to pay the electricity bill. They don't know just how bad off you are, and if they do, they have never experienced such hardship themselves and therefore can't have compassion upon you.

Let's face it, the average human is confounded by the apparently paradoxical behavior and needs of the chronically ill. Only a person who has experienced your symptoms and suffered similar hardship will be able to grasp the nuances—or blatant inconsistencies—of your behavior and offer you compassion. But even those who have "been there" cannot empathize 100% of the time, because they forget what it's like, and even they have limited capacity for pain and annoying symptoms.

What a shame that your family and friends can't adequately support you during the most trying time of your life! Yet, it's the sad reality for many and is the source of much pain and suffering for people with Lyme disease, but what's sadder is that some Lyme disease sufferers allow it to be a reason for them not to heal. They become bitter and resentful, and it consumes them. They continue to expect things that their friends and family cannot offer, including financial support, encouragement and understanding of their circumstances. Expectations keep them mired in illness and sadness.

It hurts to realize that people can't be there for us, especially those whom we most expected would be there with us through our agony.

But here's the rub. If we are to heal, then we have to let go of our expectations. We have to accept our loved ones and know that they are human, flawed and in pain, just like we are. Our suffering may be harder for them than we realize. They may want to alleviate our pain but are helpless to heal us, and that causes them anguish.

We need to focus on the good that others have given us. Recall the kind words our sisters and brothers have spoken to us, even if, in other moments, they have been cruel. Hold on to fond memories of our mothers' encouraging us, even if at times, they have chastised us for our behavior. Remember the nice evenings out which our friends paid for, even if they forgot us when we really needed help with our bills. They did the best they could, and that they have been able to do

Connie Strasheim

anything kind at all shows that they care about us, even if their capacity to give has been limited by their humanity.

Trying to see your illness from their perspective is likewise beneficial. Imagine, for example, how frustrating it must be to have to repeat the same story six times because the person you are telling it to either can't remember the details or wasn't listening to you. How difficult it must be to live with a person who suffers from bouts of depression and Lyme rage, no matter that you know that their episodes are due to Lyme disease! How taxing it must be to wonder if you are going to have to support your five kids for the rest of your life without the help of your spouse, because he or she is ill.

In my theology, only God isn't flawed. Only God can love us unconditionally. In the meantime, for the sake of your health, for the sake of learning how to give and receive love, let go of the idea that others should understand your suffering. They can't. They never will, just as sure as we can never climb into another person's soul and see their heart up close. It doesn't mean that they don't love you. They are simply human. Holding on to this realization and focusing on the good that they have given you, as well as the good that you can bring into their lives, will bring you great freedom and in turn, lighten your Lyme disease burden.

Lessons of Dating from a Disastrous Night Out

If you aren't sick enough to be housebound, but not well enough to sustain an active social life, dating can be an impractical endeavor. Knowing your limitations, expecting awkward situations on your nights out and discerning your needs, as well as your date's, can help you to determine whether or not dating will work for you. The following scenario illustrates what can happen if you end up with the wrong guy (or gal!).

Let's say Mr. Joseph Cool meets Ms. Lila Lymie at church. They strike up a conversation. From Mr. Cool's perspective, Ms. Lymie is interesting, funny and cute and he asks her out on a date. But trouble starts with the first telephone conversation, in which Ms. Lymie has forgotten half the details of their meeting arrangement, because a week has passed since that fated conversation inside of stained-glass walls.

Ms. Lymie: "Hi Joseph. I'm really looking forward to meeting you tonight. I know you've told me already, but what's the name of the restaurant where we're meeting?"

Mr. Cool: *That's strange. I thought I already told her twice?* "Little Soho. I'll see you at seven then?"

Ms. Lymie: "Sounds good...uh...just one more question, though. What kind of food do they serve at Little Soho? I mean, I know it's Japanese, but do you think I can get some vegetables there?"

(Long silence)

Mr. Cool: "I'm sure you can. Why, is there something you can't eat?"

Ms. Lymie*: Is there something I can't eat? Oh dear, where do I start? Hmmm, maybe if I just mention those things one would be likely to find at a Japanese restaurant, I'll do fine here.* "Well, I can't have white rice, or fish."

Mr. Cool: *Who doesn't eat white rice?* "You don't like fish?"

Ms. Lymie: *Now how do I tell him that I can't have fish because it's loaded with mercury and mercury makes me crazy!* "I'm allergic to it."

Mr. Cool: "Oh, okay. Maybe we should try for another kind of restaurant instead? How about Piccolo Luigi's?"

Ms. Lymie: *Italian? He's got to be joking.* Swallows hard and grips the telephone receiver. "Well, actually, I can't do pasta, either."

Connie Strasheim

Mr. Cool: *Don't tell me this is one of those high-maintenance, I can't-eat-anything, organic-food types.* "Oh, I see. Why don't you tell me what would work for you, then?"

Ms. Lymie: *What would work? I've only been asking myself that question since the onset of this dreaded illness.* "Um...well, as long as they have salad on the menu, that should be fine."

Mr. Cool: Sighs. "Okay. Well, then, how about Bennigan's?"

Ms. Lymie: *Bennigan's? Don't they use iceberg lettuce there? Couldn't he at least suggest a restaurant where salads might be a specialty? Never mind, it doesn't matter, does it? None of the restaurants in this town use organic vegetables, anyway.*
Forces enthusiasm into her voice. "Sure, why not?"

At the restaurant, Mr. Joseph Cool and Ms. Lymie sit down in a cozy booth at the back, near the bathroom.

Mr. Cool: *She's just too beautiful to be sick. Maybe she's a hypochondriac.* "Is it really true you have Lyme disease? I mean, you just look so...good!"

Ms. Lymie: Cringes. *God, how many times do I have to hear that in one day?*
Forces a smile. "Yeah, I was diagnosed two years ago."

Mr. Cool: Scrutinizes her. "So, what do you do all day long, if you aren't working? I mean, don't you get bored?"

Ms. Lymie: *Bored? If you only knew how little I get done, and how much I have to do.* "Well, healing is pretty much a full-time job."

Mr. Cool: *She's obsessed with her disorder.* Loosens his collar. "Really? Why?"

Ms. Lymie: *Must I explain coffee enemas and lymphatic drainage?* "There are just so many therapies to do."

Mr. Cool: Eyes widening in intrigue. "Oh yeah? Like what?"

Ms. Lymie: "Like coffee...I mean..." *I can't believe I almost said the word! Wonderful...maybe I should just go ahead and tell him where the rubber hose goes. That would be brilliant, wouldn't it?*

Mr. Cool: "Coffee as therapy?"

Ms. Lymie: "Well, yeah, you know, it stimulates brain circulation. I tend to have a lot of brain fog."

Mr. Cool: *Hmmm, that's strange. I could have sworn in our first conversation that she doesn't drink coffee. Oh well, must have been my imagination.*

Ms. Lymie: Fiddles with her napkin. "What did you say you do for work again? Sorry, I can't remember."

Mr. Cool: *Does she listen to a word I say?* "I'm a chemical engineer."

Ms. Lymie: Takes out a baggie of vitamin and herbal supplements. "Oh, that's right."

Mr. Cool: *She isn't really going to take all those pills before dinner, is she?* "So, uh, looks like you might need some water for those."

Ms. Lymie: Blushes. "Yeah. Do you think they have bottled water here?"

Mr. Cool: *How does this woman survive in the world?*

Ms. Lymie: *I know he's already thinking I'm a freak. If he only knew about all the pathogens and heavy metals in tap water!*

During dinner...

Connie Strasheim

Ms. Lymie: Sets down her salad fork and stands from her chair. "Excuse me, I'll be right back."

Mr. Cool: *That's the second time she's gone to the ladies' room in the last hour. I wonder what she does on long bus trips? No wait, she probably doesn't travel much, does she? Poor girl.*

Ms. Lymie: *What must he be thinking? I knew I shouldn't have accepted a date while I'm herxing. Diarrhea always shows up at the most inopportune of moments.*

After dinner, in Mr. Joseph Cool's car

Mr. Cool: "Say, what do you think about going to see that new film, Into the Wild?"

Ms. Lymie*: It's already nine p.m. If we go to a movie I won't get to bed until after midnight and then my circadian rhythm will be thrown off for a week!* "It sounds like a great flick, but I think I should be getting home now."

Mr. Cool: *Oh dear, don't tell me she's allergic to movies, too.* "Do you really need to get home now? Is there something else you'd like to do before turning in for the night?"

Ms. Lymie: Distracted. "Um, well, I don't know..." Peers under the car seat. "I think I left my scarf inside of the restaurant. I'll be right back."

Mr. Cool: "I'll wait for you here while you get it."

Ms. Lymie: Goes inside the restaurant. Returns. As she opens the passenger side door of Joseph's Honda, she forces a smile and holds up the scarf. "Left it in the bathroom. Thank goodness nobody picked it up." Drapes it around her neck and offers Joe a sheepish grin. "I really should get home now."

Mr. Cool: *Well this has been quite the night! She's a kind lady but she needs to learn how to have fun. Or does her illness just make her seem boring? Shoot, I don't know.... Maybe she does really have to have bottled water...maybe she'd go into a coma without it. What do I know? After all, I don't live inside her body. Maybe I need to give this a chance and get to know the girl behind the disease.*

Mr. Cool: "So, uh...do you want to go out again sometime?"

Ms. Lymie: Shifts in her seat. *And do what? Go to an amusement park? Get drunk at a bar? Go dancing until the wee hours of the morning? He must be kidding. I can tell he's bored. Just look at his face. I should have never accepted a date in the first place. Besides, would he pay for me every time we go out? He knows I'm not working and can barely afford groceries.*

"To be honest, Joseph, I don't see the point in us getting to know one another right now. I'm sorry, I shouldn't have accepted this date." *Then again, I had this ray of hope that you'd be different from the other guys I've met.* "Unless your idea of fun is watching an early movie or going out for organic vegetables, I'm probably not the right person for you."

Mr. Joe Cool: *Organic vegetables...early movies...and I'd probably be paying all of the time? Sighs. What a shame. Too bad she's so darned cute.* "Yeah, you know, I'm used to going out on the weekend and living a little. I need that after a hard week at work. I'd love to go out again, but I'm not sure what that would look like. After all, it seems you can't go to many restaurants, and since I don't get off work until six, that gets me to your place by seven. An evening that ends at nine o'clock just isn't much of an evening, you know?"

Ms. Lymie: *It'll just be easier if I do my own thing. I can't start eating pasta and screwing up my health for a man. Besides, he doesn't understand what Lyme disease can do to a person's emotions. No, it's not really worth it.* She buttons up her coat and sighs. "Yes, I know what you mean, and it's okay. It's been really nice getting to know you, though. Thanks for the, uh—interesting evening."

Connie Strasheim

Chapter 11

Finances and Work

No Dough to Throw at Lyme Disease: Formulating a Protocol on a Shoestring Budget

Does your kitchen look like a pharmacy? Do you routinely try new supplements in an attempt to accommodate your symptom picture? Are you able to purchase new products at whim in order to aid in your bug-killing and nutritional protocol? If you answered "yes" to any of the above questions, chances are, you have the financial resources to build a hefty arsenal against Borrelia and the Co-Infection Company.

But what if you can't work and don't have family or friends to provide for you? What can you do to get rid of Lyme disease if you don't have a nice fistful of batter to make yourself a triple-layer treatment cake?

Strategic choices when putting together a Lyme disease treatment plan can enable you to battle illness without spending much money. Following is an example of an inexpensive protocol that addresses the three vital components of healing, which include: 1) infection eradication, 2) supporting the body's nutritional needs and 3) detoxifying

Connie Strasheim

organs and tissues. I wish I could say that the following plan is adequate for all, but there's no one-size-fits-all strategy when it comes to treating Lyme disease. It is, however, a good start that can bring you one step closer to remission, and if you're lucky, may be enough to finish the battle for you. The components and details of this treatment plan have been discussed earlier in the book.

1. First, you'll need something to kill the critters. Taking a quality sea salt such as Redmond's, along with high doses of Vitamin C has been shown, in some cases, to be sufficient for combating Lyme disease and co-infections. Check out: www.lymephotos.com and www.fettnet.com/lymestrategies/welcome.htm for information on how to do this protocol. Another option is MMS, Miracle Mineral Supplement. This therapy has not been tested at length in chronic Lyme disease sufferers but it has allegedly cured thousands of malaria and other illnesses and its preliminary results in Lyme disease patients have been excellent. One physician who is using this product has stated that the results of MMS on his patients have been better than pharmaceutical antibiotics. For more information, check out: www.miraclemineral.org. At less than fifty dollars a month, salt/C and MMS cost only a fraction of other treatments, such as antibiotics and herbs.

2. Lyme disease is a pro at creating nutritional deficiencies and biochemical dysfunction, so you'll want to purchase a good food-based multi-vitamin, magnesium, trace minerals, fish oil and perhaps a probiotic and/or digestive enzymes. These five or six items will provide much of the supplemental nutrition that your body needs to help battle infections and keep its systems functioning properly. If you cannot afford all of these supplements, then ensure that your diet includes a high nutritional intake of all of the above from food sources, preferably organic.

3. Finally, you'll want to do something to get all those toxins that dying bugs produce out of your body. Great kidney, lymph, blood and liver detoxification protocols can be prepared using

mostly fresh foods rather than costly drugs or herbal combinations. Juicing fruits and raw vegetables is especially beneficial. For instance, a juice prepared with beets, cucumbers and carrots is great for cleansing the liver and gall bladder, while cranberry juice, parsley and asparagus are good for the kidneys and bladder. One additional and helpful purchase is an enema bag, to perform coffee enemas. Enemas detoxify the colon and liver and can be bought at Wal-Mart for $5.00.

To Get a Job or Not Get a Job

How often do you ask yourself if you are able to work? Especially when you awaken one day feeling almost normal but on the next, you have a body that feels about as stable as a boneless chicken, with a foggy brain to boot.

Your friends and family suggest you get a job. After all, you did go dancing last weekend, didn't you? But you, and they, conveniently forget about the post-exertional malaise that greeted you the following morning when you parted from your bed sheets.

Yet on that almost normal day, you think, "Hey, I've got energy today! Maybe I'll do ten loads of laundry, send out fifty resumés and then after breakfast, call a couple hundred employers!"

If you're like me, you'll feel guilty if, on days like this, you don't at least conceive of productivity, but I'm also learning that it's not always good to whip out the Super Girl hose when you kinda, sorta feel good.

At one point during my second year of being really ill with Lyme disease, my symptoms abated, and I decided to work part-time as a medical interpreter for Spanish-speaking patients. I thought, What better job than to do something I enjoyed, and for just a few hours here and there? Besides, it would take my mind off my illness, right?

Wrong. My attempt to jump back into the "real world" left me flattened as I discovered that any appointment before noon wreaked

Connie Strasheim

havoc with my circadian rhythm, as the anticipation of having to get up by a certain time ensured that I didn't sleep well. Brain fog made it difficult for me to concentrate during crucial moments, and driving from clinic to clinic in crazy traffic sucked up more adrenaline than I had in reserves, as did dealing with impatient doctors and fearful patients. On top of it all, my boss had anger and memory problems and was prone to random outbursts and not paying her interpreters for their work. (Maybe she had Lyme disease, eh?) The cherry on the cake of inconveniences was that I no longer had as much time as before to dedicate to my healing.

Since then, I've thought about employment again. Every day when my energy meter climbs into the green and I look at my sorry bank account, I conceive of putting on some Superwoman spandex again. But then I recall my experience two years ago and reconsider. On many days, I feel seventy or eighty percent healed from this illness, but I've learned that this percentage must remain constant if I hope to work full-time. It's important to take the consistency factor into consideration on days when you feel good. Do you feel decent enough to work on most days? How about eighty percent of the time? Much less than that and you will struggle in a job.

Sadly, some people with Lyme disease don't have a choice when it comes to employment. If you have children to support or don't have relatives to care for you, you work or else beg on a corner and lose the roof over your head. Some Lymefolk take harmful doses of steroids or other medications in order to be able to work, and for them, it's the only way out. Others suffer tremendously under the burden of having to work. Many take naps during their lunch hour, come home from their jobs, have dinner, and then sleep for twelve hours before getting up to do it all over again. For others who have family to partially support them, the option of being able to take time off to dedicate to their healing is a possibility, if not a necessity.

In the end, the question may be, is it a greater stress for you to work or to struggle financially? Will you have time to dedicate to your Lyme disease treatments if you work full-time? Will your healing be hindered by the physical and mental demands of work? Or will you feel helpless and depressed if you can't get out of the house?

If you are led to stay home and take care of yourself, don't feel guilty! Sometimes healing is a full-time job, even if you are able to go out and salsa sometimes on Saturday night. Or if you've had a string of good weeks or months, then why not try on the suit of employment? Put it on slowly, however, to make sure it fits where you are at in your healing journey. Sometimes, you can't know until you get out there whether employment is for now or another time.

Connie Strasheim

Chapter 12

Travel

Tips for Airplane Travel when You're Symptomatic

You toss and turn in bed, envisioning tomorrow's nightmare travel day. Do you really want to get on an airplane again? You know you need a vacation; you have spent the last two years of your life house-bound with Lyme disease. But you've traveled enough in the past to know what awaits you as you prepare to transport your body across the United States, and you're not sure that you can do this.

You can see it now. It all starts as you wait in line at the check-in counter with screaming children, irritable airline employees and a thousand perfumes to pulverize your immune system. Then your postural-orthostatic-tachycardia syndrome kicks in as you stand, lugging a one-hundred-pound suitcase behind you and a backpack that isn't much lighter, up to the check-in counter.

You envision the tired attendant snapping your head off when you ask for an exit row on the five-hour flight to San Diego. Nope, it'll be a middle seat in row 38 on a Boeing 777. Your restlessness increases as you picture the security line winding halfway around the airport and

Connie Strasheim

TSA personnel tossing out two-thirds of the contents of your carry-on bag.

You'll be wasted by the time you get to the gate, never mind the flight to San Diego. You ask yourself again whether this sabbatical is worth it. If you have to sit in 38E, that means any number of annoyances could sit on either side of you. A traveler wearing perfume, another who spills his weight onto your side of the armrest. Not to mention the kid in front of you who reclines his seat for all but take-off and landing. You'll get a blood clot in your leg for sure. Should you spend extra money for an upgrade?

You sigh and flip over in bed. What will you do with your suitcase when you get to the airport? You don't really want to check it, but unless the passenger standing behind you on the airplane helps you to haul it into the overhead bin, you won't be able to take the thing onboard with you because you'll be too weak to lift it.

And what about the dehydration factor? You know you won't get enough to drink on the plane because the flight attendants have enough to do without you asking them for a beverage every half-hour. Your best friend is a flight attendant, you know how overworked they are, and you'll feel guilty if you need to ask for a drink five times during the flight.

Your mind wanders to thoughts of stinky lavatories, the lack of space aboard the aircraft, recycled air and no medical care. Oh dear. What if your air hunger gets out of control? Are you really well enough to travel?

Airplane travel can be a frustrating experience for the well-seasoned, healthy traveler, and a downright nightmare for those with Lyme disease. Before you decide whether it's worth enduring, consider that your ability to travel will depend upon your specific needs and limitations, as well as how well-informed you are about the procedures and potential difficulties of airplane travel. Often, it's not as much a matter of your energy or pain level as it is your inability to stand or your allergies and chemical sensitivities, and while you can't do anything about these challenges, you can take steps to make air travel easier.

I've been fortunate to be able to travel on airplanes despite having Lyme disease, even during times when I've been quite sick. Having been a flight attendant for eight years means that I know exactly what I need to do in order to travel with minimum stress. While jet lag, jet fuel and long lines exhaust me, too, it's because I know how things work that I can mostly relax when I get to the airport, which saves me a ton of energy.

I surmise that one of the biggest reasons why air travel is exhausting is because of the emotional stress. Forget jet lag and long flights. Often, it's all about the adrenaline and fear sensations that people associate with air travel, and it all starts in bed. You set four alarm clocks but don't sleep anyway for fear of missing your flight, as if it were a life and death situation if the airplane left without you! Then you underestimate the time it takes to put the finishing touches on your packing and haul two large suitcases out to the car, and fret when these add ten unanticipated extra minutes to your morning get-ready time. You skip breakfast because you want to make sure you make it to the airport, and you head out, groggy, rushed and hungry. The worry mounts when you find yourself stuck in traffic at seven a.m., and is exacerbated when the airport shuttle takes twenty minutes before it picks you up to take you to the terminal building—and that's just the beginning!

The long check-in lines leave you wondering if you'll miss your flight and airport security violates your privacy by displaying your underwear all over their inspection tables. You sweat inside the terminal as you scurry to purchase water and use the toilet before boarding the plane. At the gate, you bite your nails wondering if you'll get your upgrade or at least an aisle seat. You grumble over how long it takes for people to board the airplane, fret over the lack of overhead space, then, once seated, worry when the captain announces that there's a mechanical problem with the airplane! It's never-ending. Never mind the airplane inconveniences: small seats, crying babies, not enough to drink, no place to put your briefcase or your legs...you get the point.

Connie Strasheim

How can you avoid such stress, short of taking a sedative? Not that there's anything wrong with taking a sedative. If that's what it takes, then by all means, take a mind relaxant and save your poor adrenal glands the work of secreting excess adrenaline. They need that to fight Lyme disease, not to make sure you get on your airplane.

Following are some tips that can help to make air travel easier, or simply possible, when you have Lyme disease.

1. Allow yourself an extra half-hour in the morning for a good protein and carbohydrate breakfast and any last-minute packing.

2. If you're going to lose sleep over missing your flight, then take a sedative for this, too. Tell yourself it's better to miss your flight than to tax your body with worry.

3. Sit on your luggage while waiting in the check-in line to conserve energy, and browse a magazine. Waiting and anticipation are stressful.

4. If you end up getting a middle seat in the back of the Economy cabin, tell yourself you'll get up often during the flight and make best friends with your flight companions. If you sit next to someone wearing perfume, ask someone else to switch seats with you.

5. Anticipate how long airline shuttles can take. Anticipate all kinds of delays but don't stress over them.

6. Consider that airport Security is going to poke around in your personal belongings and leave the scary stuff at the bottom of your suitcase.

7. Bring earplugs to drown out the screaming kids, a blow-up pillow to rest your head against so you can doze, and ibuprofen and aspirin in case the earplugs don't work. If you forget your

meds, flight attendants on most airlines carry aspirin and ace-taminophen (Tylenol). Tell yourself that you don't have to hurry. Again and again and again!

8. If you need to frequent the toilet during flight, ask for an aisle seat. If none are available, then you might want to tell the person sitting next to you that you'll have to get up often during the flight. If you feel bad about having to say this, don't! Your needs are just as important as anyone else's. I had to do this on a flight to Australia, and I found my seat companions to be very understanding. You can also ask someone else to switch seats with you so that you can sit in the aisle. If you are lucky, you may be able to request a bulk head or an exit row seat, which usually offer plenty of space for getting up and moving past others who are sitting in your row, not to mention extra leg room.

9. Make sure you drink enough water by bringing an empty bottle from home to fill in the airport terminal or on the airplane. This can make a huge difference in your travel experience, as airplanes are extremely dehydrating. Bring a large, two-liter bottle for international flights and at least a liter for a domestic flight. Bring a larger bottle if your itinerary involves two or more flights, as wait time in-between makes for a long travel day.

10. Bring food from home. Many Lyme disease sufferers consume healthy, organic food, which is impossible to find in airports. A chicken or tuna salad in a plastic container, along with other snacks, such as fruit, nuts and cheese, can keep your mood and blood sugar stable. Waiting in-between flights means that your travel day can end up being long, so pack as much food as you can carry without becoming overburdened with weight. If you don't want to bother with food preparation or lugging around the extra weight of food, at least consider some nuts or string cheese. You never know when you'll be caught in a three-hour delay on the runway.

Connie Strasheim

11. If you have problems standing in line, consider getting a doctor's note in order to bypass long security and check-in lines.

12. Temperatures on airplanes and in gate areas fluctuate. Dress in layers. Leave the heavy coat behind and opt for a lighter jacket, with a wool sweater and/or tee shirt beneath. Wear sturdy, comfortable walking shoes and don't take anything in your carry-on luggage that you don't absolutely need for the flight. At the same time, make sure you carry medications and any other essentials with you, just in case your checked luggage doesn't make it with you on time to your final destination.

13. Bring a couple of paperback books or puzzles so that you have something to do while waiting in gate areas and on the airplane. Take some lighter reading that will make sense even after you've been airborne for two hours and hypoxia (oxygen deprivation) starts to set in. Music can be nice to have along, too, as long as it doesn't add too much weight to your pack.

If you're concerned about having a medical emergency onboard your flight, you should know that there is usually a passenger on most flights who is a medical professional of some sort: a physician, nurse or EMT. As well, flight attendants have basic knowledge of medical care, CPR training and AED defibrillator training. The airplane cockpit contains an emergency medical kit that is designed for use by health care practitioners. If you feel nauseous, light-headed or weak, supplemental oxygen is also available on all airplanes. In cases of emergency, pilots can divert to nearby airports. During my eight years as a flight attendant, I never witnessed a single medical emergency onboard that could not be resolved with the means available to the flight crew.

Finally, I believe that some of the "What-if?" thinking that occurs in people with Lyme disease may have more to do with the unfamiliarity of travel and less to do with worry about whether Lyme disease symptoms will prevent them from traveling or getting on an airplane. Yes, an emergency could occur while you are overseas in Thailand, and yes, you could pass out on the airplane. Chances are, however, if you are able to move about in your own city and can be in public places, you can probably travel to at least some destinations. If you haven't boarded an airplane in a long time, doing a short trip with a companion is a good way to test your ability to fly.

Be prudent and take care of your body. Airplane travel is taxing, even for those who aren't ill. On the other hand, I wouldn't recommend insulating yourself from it based on a few "What if's?." Part of healing involves taking risks. There is much joy and freedom in being able to leave home, and if you are fortunate enough to be able to get around in public places, you may be surprised at how well you fare traveling.

Connie Strasheim

Chapter 13

Helping Others

We All Advocate what Works for Us: Taking Care when Leading Another Towards Health

When it comes to my friend Lokie the Lymie, I just can't take off my white lab coat and refrain from suggesting a half-dozen remedies to fix my poor, busted-up friend, no matter that I know nothing about what he really needs.

I've had over three years to learn about Lyme disease, but the more I feed my brain with knowledge, the more I realize that I don't know green squash about this illness and the human body. I might have bits n' pieces of useful knowledge to offer my ailing friend, but it's biased, based on my personal experience and the few dozen books I've read, and so I urge Lokie to try the remedies that have worked for me—when Lokie probably really needs something else.

Shouldn't we all share what we've learned about Lyme disease in order to help others? Of course! We do a disservice to them if we don't. Yet even the best of healers can't know what treatment protocol will put a person into remission, because we are all unique and there's no one-size-fits-all remedy when it comes to this disease. Hence, we ought to

Connie Strasheim

tread carefully before insisting that we know what will work for another. Consider that if borrelia is a complicated organism, how much more is the human body!

We have been to the moon, made airplanes and created the Internet, but know close to *nada* about our biochemistry. Our cells carry out extraordinarily complex tasks without us knowing the how or why of it all. We are the machine, but we don't know what makes us stop or start. We can't push our own biochemical buttons, much less find the ones needing repair, because the missing part is itty bitty and not the one we think we need. It's not even a piece that will work on other machines.

Fortunately, we've been given clues to help us fix the machinery that's been fouled up by Lyme disease. But where we have been allowed to make discoveries, we soon learn that this is all they are; revelations that add another piece to the puzzle, perhaps not even our own, and which are seldom a panacea.

But that's okay, because if we allow them to, clues keep us from the arrogant notion that the therapies that have cured us from Lyme disease should always and absolutely work for Lokie and others we know. They keep us from being pushy in our views and from believing that we have the one and only answer to the problem of borrelia. Realizing that we own little pieces, instead of the whole puzzle, is the first step towards effectively using what Lyme disease has taught us, in order to help others heal as they fit their pieces with ours.

Energy and Spoons: Chronic Fatigue Sufferers Don't Get Much Silverware

Many sufferers of chronic fatigue are familiar with the spoon theory, an analogy that measures daily energy reserves in terms of spoons. The average healthy person might get, say, fifty spoons a day, while a chronic fatigue sufferer gets only twenty, or thirty. I don't know why spoons were decided upon as the symbol for energy reserves. Why not forks, or knives? How about a points system?

Anyway, following is my adapted application of the spoon theory at work, which you can show your friends and family members who don't understand why you won't just pull your arse out of the armchair and get a job like the rest of the world. They still won't know what you are going through—no soul who hasn't suffered from chronic illness ever can—but this analogy will give them a glimpse into a life that otherwise baffles them.

Before you were sick, let's suppose that you had fifty sterling spoons in your energy drawer. Now that you have chronic fatigue, twenty-five of those pieces are in the dishwasher, and nobody's unloaded it for eons. So you have twenty-five spoons left in your drawer, which get used, re-washed and put back into the drawer every day or every other day. Each daily activity costs you some spoons, and your activities are more costly than your healthy friend Bouncer's, who not only has a drawer full of fifty-plus spoons but who also seems to get more use out of his.

You can do just about anything that Bouncer can, if you're willing to give up your spoons. You can accompany him for an hour-long run, but you might as well toss your entire twenty-five spoons for the next two days into the dishwasher, while Bouncer only throws in ten of his to complete the task.

You have to choose your activities wisely, and you're a little jealous of Bouncer.

Being so shortchanged on silverware, you've also grown keen to the fact that emotional, mental and physical energy aren't created equally, and that emotional energy is often the most costly. When you had health like Bouncer's, you were too blind to notice this. You took it for granted. Now, even if you do nothing but lie in bed all day, if your emotions are a mess, then all of your spoons are filthy and your energy drawer is almost empty. When you were healthier, you would have never noticed this to be true, but even in illness, there are times when you don't realize that you've used up all your spoons until it's time for another meal. Then you have to spend a day on the sofa while your spoons get cleaned and Bouncer takes care of you.

Connie Strasheim

There is a positive side to having fewer spoons than when you were in sterling health (besides being taken care of by Bouncer!). You cherish and appreciate your spoons more than when they were spilling over the edges of your energy drawer, and you stay away from activities that drain you, because you just can't afford to waste your precious silver. If you retain this appreciation, perhaps once you are healed, you'll never let the dishwasher get completely full again. In the meantime, you hope that your friends and family understand when, after long dinners at your house, you don't have any spoons leftover for ice-cream.

Chapter 14

Habits

Keeping a Lyme Log to Track Your Progress

Maybe you're not into journaling or jotting down your daily agonies, but have you ever considered keeping a log of your Lyme disease symptoms and treatments, for the sake of tracking your progress and honing your protocol? If not a daily one, then how about a weekly, or monthly one?

If your mind is like mine, then it often operates on fuzz and buzz mode, which makes memory unreliable for recalling past symptoms and knowledge of what treatments have or haven't worked for you. Also, trying to assess progress without use of a written history for comparison is to rely upon a mind filled with biases and that's subject to poor interpretations of past experiences. When brain fog or depression are strong, you really can't trust your thoughts! Additionally, if you frequently change your protocol, you may miss or misunderstand the effects of a treatment upon your body. Keeping a log can help you to correlate symptoms with treatments in a more detailed, accurate way.

Connie Strasheim

It doesn't have to be tedious. If you are lazy or undisciplined or really ill, how about just writing a brief summary once a month? You can put a sticky note on your bathroom mirror or on your forehead (just kidding) to remind you on what date you're supposed do this.

Making detailed notes regarding how and when symptoms occur can be important. If fuzz and buzz prohibit you from recalling details, then you'll have to settle for the less effective method of vague interpretations, or else make it a habit to jot down symptoms on a more regular basis.

Bear in mind that subtle changes in healing can be missed when you use generic terms to describe your symptoms and under what circumstances they occur. For instance, writing, 'Fatigue and brain fog in the morning until 11:00 A.M. prevents me from reading,' is much more descriptive than writing, 'Today, I have bad fatigue and brain fog.' Specific details allow you to recognize progress when, a year later, you still have 'bad fatigue and brain fog' but you are now able to read in the morning by 9:00 A.M. instead of 11:00 A.M.

Correlating treatments with progress can be more difficult, especially if you are doing multiple protocols simultaneously. Still, it can be useful to keep a record of your treatments, particularly supplements, and the changes you experience hours, days or weeks after starting or stopping them.

If you don't like to write long paragraphs, doing a graph with columns and rows is another way to track progress. Or train yourself to use abbreviations (although personally, that would be too tedious for my Lyme brain!).

I didn't start keeping a log until one year into my illness, and even then, it was a monthly summary that provided few details on my symptoms and healing strategies. More than once I've wished that I could better recall how I felt in previous months and how different supplements affected me. As of late I've started a weekly log, and I spend just five minutes at the end of each week scrawling out my thoughts. I stick the notebook bedside, where I know I won't forget it!

I encourage you to do the same. At least try it for a few months and see if it proves to be helpful for discerning progress and for determining which strategies are working for you.

The Problem with, and Usefulness of, "To-Do" Lists

Have you ever found that "To-Do" lists can provide you with vital instructions on what to do with yourself each day? If you are like me, you find that brain fog and an open schedule leave you prone to fiddling around and wasting time, and that having an agenda can help you to focus and use your time wisely.

Before I go to bed, I scrawl out ten or fifteen things that I hope to accomplish the following day. If I didn't do this, I'd spend the first half of my day just trying to get my sluggish self together, and by nightfall, thoughts of, "I- shoulda-coulda-done-this-or-that" would be floating through my head. Ah, the bedtime recriminations, which are so unhealthy for a Lyme disease sufferer! Hence, the "To-Do" list allows me to sleep confidently, by telling me what to do with my wandering energies upon arising in the morning.

Problem is, I tend to forget that I have Lyme disease when I compile the list of what I need to do the following day, and end up making an agenda better suited for Superwoman. Sometimes, I catch myself in the act, but justify the two thousand activities by telling myself, "just in case you have extra time, you'll have something else to catch up on." When do I ever have extra time? When do I finish the "To-Do" list with time to spare? Never! Don't fall into this trap, or you may find yourself under pressure to get more done than you should. You don't want the thing that's intended to reduce your daily stress levels to put you in fast-forward mode as you strive to accomplish all the daily goals that you set for yourself. Make a list, but don't make it too long, and let some of it go if you have a symptom flare day and end up not being able to do much. Don't worry about the laundry. You can probably make do with another day in the same shirt.

Connie Strasheim

I'm learning that cutting my daily responsibilities down to size is a crucial step in my healing process. The "To-Do" list can be beneficial, but if not used wisely can also create pressure to perform, which is an immense stress on the body. Yet, it remains a useful tool for my tired existence, and it may be for you too, as long as it helps to keep you focused and productive, and you can discern when enough is enough.

The Dangers of Leading a High Cortisol Lifestyle

The western world is becoming prey to what I call the high cortisol lifestyle, and I surmise that it's part of the reason why chronic illness is on the rise in places such as the United States, Canada, Europe and Australia. Cortisol is a hormone secreted by the adrenal glands, those itsy-bitsy triangular glands that sit atop the kidneys. Cortisol is responsible, along with other hormones, for a multitude of bodily functions, including blood sugar and blood pressure regulation, fighting inflammation, mobilizing energy for the brain and enabling the body to deal with stress, whether it be emotional, nutritional, physiological or hormonal.

Stress is a normal part of life, but did you know that the western world's ways are conducive to adrenal fatigue and illness, as a result of excessive demands put on the adrenal glands to produce cortisol?

We thrive on stimulus. Without it, we are bored. Stimulus from the Internet, stimulus from recreational activities and stimulus all day long because we need to occupy our minds and bodies 24-7. We eat fast, drive fast, talk fast and constantly check our watches to ensure that we aren't going to be late for the next stressful, harrying event.

The adrenals often don't have the capacity to meet the demands we place upon them, as such stimuli require more biochemicals than our bodies can produce. Who knows, maybe the adrenals would be able to cope if fed a proper diet and provided with proper rest amidst the frenzy?

Unfortunately, the rush-hurry-need-more-of-this lifestyle means that we won't take the time to prepare a home-cooked meal with healthy, fresh ingredients, and especially not three times a day! We opt instead for the nutrient-less, imitation food in a box or poison fast food burgers and so deprive our adrenal glands of the raw materials they need to produce the proper amount of biochemicals so that we can continue on with our frenzy.

No, the stimulus lifestyle is just too addicting and shutting off the race-race mentality after a long day at work is never an option, and so we cram recreation and ten thousand best friends into our off-hours. And as for going to bed early and getting a good eight hours of rest? I don't think so!

Gosh, those adrenal glands are just so tiny. Were they really meant to work that hard?

What can we do? Would any of us ever consider cutting activities from our lives in order to give our adrenals a break, especially now that we have Lyme disease?

Would we consider changing our diets, though it would mean not going out to lunch with co-workers? Could we leave some of our daily activities for tomorrow's "to do" list?

Should we risk getting screamed at, or fired, from work because we want to accomplish tasks at a healthier pace? Is our health worth it? Would we be willing to lose the Mr. Popularity award by giving up activities with friends when we're exhausted? Could we go to bed an hour earlier and give up Jay Leno?

Hmmm...

Our bodies need stress in the proper amounts, or things will start to go wrong. If you are suffering from symptoms of the high cortisol lifestyle, you'll need to slow down so that your immune system can be strong enough to fight Lyme disease. So chew that salmon steak fifty times, spend a day without your watch and forgo the fast lane! Just

Connie Strasheim

because you are sick doesn't mean you should try to make up for lost time by cramming more activities into your life at times when you feel good. If you want to recover, you must let go of the need to move fast and be productive.

Chapter 15

For the Day-to-Day

Must Your Life Be All About Lyme Disease? Ways to Get Out of Your Head

How is it possible that at least every other thought I have is, in some way, related to Lyme disease?

I often chastise myself for having a brain full of borrelia bits, because life is more than this dastardly illness, but how difficult it is to live out this truth when my minutes are filled with little reminders from my body that I do, in fact, have Lyme disease. Even if I ceased to write about Lyme, stayed away from the support groups and stopped all of my treatments, I surmise that I'd remain mired in thoughts of illness because every two minutes I feel how broken I am!

Yet, something about devoting a huge percentage of my thoughts to this illness scares me. Do you know what I mean? Not that we shouldn't do all that is within our power to heal, but is it possible—and I'm about to say something bold here—that some of us stay sick because thoughts of disease and how to heal the body occupy too much brain space?

Connie Strasheim

I wouldn't blame you for leasing out your mind to Lyme disease. Chronic illness has a way of screaming for your undivided attention, and healing is often a tremendous investment of energy and resources. How can you not think about it?

But here's the rub. Life is so much larger than what we suffer and our attempts to fix it, and I'm not convinced that giving Lyme disease my near-undivided attention is the way out. No matter how much I tell myself that I need to research cat's claw or spend two hours daily doing cognitive therapy and another two getting answers and encouragement on an Internet Yahoo! support group.

I think some of my thoughts need to be diverted to the world and its needs. I'm not denying the adage that we can't help others until we help ourselves. It is true that you can't give to the world when you don't have anything to give away, but are there any of us who are that broken? We don't need to volunteer at the local Red Cross or do some great humanitarian act of service, but getting involved in the world in small, positive ways can be an excellent way to promote healing by getting us out of our own heads.

By painting greeting cards, for example. Or becoming an on-line advocate for abolishing war in Sudan. Or how about gardening, making CD's for a friend, or starting a scrapbook? Just doing something, anything, that contributes positively to the world and which steers your synapses away from Lyme disease.

So why not? Well...some of us just don't feel like doing other things. We're tired, and fear keeps us rooted in all things Lyme. As long as there is research to be done, or a new symptom clamoring for relief, we won't want to give other things in life an iota of our attention. For me, I prefer the excuse that much of what I know these days is about Lyme disease, and I should use that knowledge to help others.

For the sake of your healing, however, try another science experiment. Forget your aches, forget the next Lyme book you need to read and instead pick up a novel.

You may wonder how it's possible to give the brain another hobby when life's circumstances conspire to suck you into thoughts of disease and worries about how to fix your broken body. Shouldn't you make it your life's mission to heal? After all, without your physical health, you don't have anything, right?

Consider that healing might instead be achieved when you open your life to something greater than fixing what ails you, but not to the exclusion of caring for yourself. Perhaps it involves acknowledging and trusting your creator to guide you in the best way to spend your time and energy, as you release the fears that keep you entrenched in musings of illness.

For me, it is an act of the will and asking God every day to nudge me in the right direction and then believing that the best thing will be done for me.

And I have found that, whenever I am able to pull myself away from thoughts of Lyme disease by engaging in other activities, I feel more balanced and at peace.

Recently, a friend and fellow Lyme disease sufferer wrote to me about how getting a job had proved to be more healing for her than staying at home, despite the physical challenges of work, because she was able to get out of her "Lyme brain."

Not all of us with Lyme disease are healthy enough to work, but where the line seems to be blurred, why not try a paid activity or volunteer job doing research for a worthy cause? (Besides Lyme disease!) Doing this, or some other meaningful brain diversion, could give your immune system a boost in ways you hadn't thought possible.

Energy versus Hyperactivity and Learning to Slow Down

Before I had severe symptoms of Lyme disease, I was the Queen of High Speed. Electric and lit like a thousand-watt bulb. Just plug me in

Connie Strasheim

and watch me go! Moving, fast, full speed ahead, a super comet, super woman until...Boom! I'd crash.

Now, even though I have less energy than before becoming seriously ill in 2004, on a good day, I still bounce around the house like the energizer bunny, then jump into my hamster wheel and go, go, go! Hurry, faster, faster! And I still crash, but harder now. No, I haven't learned my lesson.

I doubt I'm alone in this. You know how great it feels when you get a burst of energy. You just can't help but be an adrenaline junkie when your cells get an extra shot of ATP, even though a voice is hissing inside of your head, "This is part of the reason you're in the fix of chronic illness!" No, you want to take advantage of that energy and get things done!

I'm starting to realize, however, that my energy isn't just the result of a societal pull to do things ever faster and with greater efficiency. It's also a Lyme disease symptom, and its name is hyperactivity. It's not real energy, but a force that compels me to go, go, go and do life at a breakneck speed before crashing and burning.

I'm convinced we can take life slower. Yes, we can beat society and those borrelia buggers who plug us into a socket and keep us wired but tired all day, but it requires mindfulness. An awareness of when we are eating too fast, talking too fast, or dashing about the house from one room to another, trying to complete a million tasks in an hour. It requires stopping and heeding the voice within that's warning us of an impending crash. It's realizing that the world won't end if we sit on the sofa and do nothing. It's spending time in prayer and meditation, to get centered and to develop an awareness of other things in life besides our to-do lists.

While it may be difficult at first to slow down, especially if a bunch of bugs are conspiring to push your buttons, consider that heeding the hyperactive trigger, or allowing yourself to operate on fast forward every time you get a spurt of energy, isn't beneficial to the body. In fact, too much adrenaline breaks down the immune system. When you rest, your body heals. When you rush, your body struggles. It's that simple.

The Necessity of a Multi-faceted Approach to Healing

Lyme disease and its co-infections are special little suckers. Unlike the treatment of other pathogens, they demand your undivided attention due to the mess they make of your body. There's always so much clean-up and trying to get things back in order, because the pathogens party hard and invite two thousand of their closest infectious friends over whenever possible, as they tear down the house that is your body.

I can just hear them now, "Hey Herpes! The immune system's out! Come on over!"

The implication of this is that you can't just take a few antibiotics and hope for the best. These bugs are tenacious and intelligent. A multi-faceted approach to healing is therefore important and should include:

1. Killing borrelia and its co-infections, whether babesia, candida, mold or monkey pox virus (just kidding on that last one). Just pick your favorite pathogen and go to it.

2. Doing something with all of that bug die-off. Get it out of the body! Make your new mantra, detox, detox, detox! Chlorella, French green clay (yes, you can eat clay), cholestyramine, mucuna bean powder, zeolites, ionic foot baths, detox foot pads, as well as strategies mentioned in earlier chapters, are some good ways to remove toxins from the body.

3. Keeping the organs and body systems functioning smoothly amidst all the killing and toxin mop-up. A healthy, balanced diet, along with herbal, vitamin and hormonal supplements can assist with this. Try some iodine for the thyroid, Siberian ginseng and licorice for the adrenal glands, beets for the liver and fish oil for the brain, for example.

Connie Strasheim

4. Staying spiritual. Listen to God and spend time in prayer and contemplation. Believe in your body's ability to heal. Don't overlook the emotional aspect of healing. Doing this will give you better results with all of the aforementioned.

The Power of Environment to Heal

Have you ever wondered if changing your environment could help you to heal?

I live in a relatively polluted, high-altitude city and used to ask myself this question, thinking that a change of climate and city would accelerate my healing process. One day, I managed to schlep my body south to Costa Rica for five weeks, to test this hypothesis, and found that indeed, climate, as well as the pollution level of a city or town, affected my symptoms. I felt stellar in the rainforest and less functional in the contaminated capital of San Jose or in areas where it was hot and muggy.

At the same time, I was reminded that there's more to one's healing environment than just climate and level of pollution. Whenever a smiling local would help me with my luggage, or I shared a relaxed meal with expatriates or observed the non-hurried, polite manner of a cashier, I felt at ease myself, and my symptoms seemed to abate.

Expatriates and locals told me that many foreigners who come to Costa Rica never leave, and not just because of the weather, gorgeous greenery and slightly lower cost of living. They stay because of the ready smiles, the laid-back way of life, and tranquil, hospitable manner of the locals. They stay because they can arrive at work at eight-fifteen and nobody is going to scream at them for being late. They stay because they know that if they were to fall and scrape their leg on the sidewalk, a half-dozen others would rush to their aid. They stay because life isn´t "just about me," but also the community. If your neighbor needs help mending his fence, you help him. It's a done deed. And if you ask a Costa Rican where the supermarket is, she´ll often walk you there, no matter that she's in the middle of cooking her children breakfast.

Expatriates also stay because losing a lifetime of material possessions actually gives them one less thing to worry about and because the philosophy of the people is that while life is hard, it's okay. In the end, it all works out. Many believe that it is God who owns everything and is in control; there are fish in the sea and bananas on the trees, so why fret?

Yes, sometimes the *ticos*, as the locals are called, fake a smile when they would rather scream. Or so I've heard, but if you don't know that, it doesn't matter because the smile is there all the same.

Could such a mindset of tranquility, of open generosity, and an attitude that is mindful of the well-being of others be part of why folks from overseas find healing here, and why Costa Rica ranks high on the list of the world's healthiest countries to live in?

Of course, people everywhere have the capacity to give and receive love. In Costa Rica, however, it seems to be built into the cultural norms in such a way that promotes health and attracts others to its shores.

Could I heal of Lyme disease by thinking more about the man at the church begging for a few colones? Would I recover faster if I let it be no big deal that I just missed the bus and got soaked in the rain? Would my body thank me for lunches that are a bit more leisurely?

While most of us can't experiment with living overseas, we can influence our environment at home. Where there is strife, hurry and stress, we should do all that is within our power to change that situation. Where there is pollution and limited access to fresh food and a healthy community of friends, we ought to move. And whenever we jump on a negative train over trivialities and inconveniences, we should remind ourselves to get off at the next stop, because not everything in life should be treated as though it were an emergency.

Connie Strasheim

Taking a Vacation from Illness to Enjoy Life

I've been blessed to have airline travel benefits over the past few years while sick with Lyme disease. Travel has been such medicine to my soul that, whether half-dead or sorta thriving, whether broke or with a few bucks in my pocket, I manage to haul my body overseas at least a couple of times a year. I just have to, even though travel is physically difficult for me.

The distraction of exotic cultures and environments infuse my spirit with life, partly because they enable me to take a vacation from Lyme disease and all of its accompanying worries. While I continue to experience symptoms whenever I travel, they tend to be submerged beneath the excitement of being in a new place.

Why, just sitting in a plaza surrounded by ancient architecture, or having an intriguing conversation with a local, removes me from thoughts of wondering how I'll pay for my mortgage next month, or how many pills I'll have to order tomorrow. No hamster wheel of treatments, no pressuring myself to hurry up and find the right protocol so I can heal and get out into the working world again.

And, since it's impossible for me to adhere to my Lyme diet overseas, I get to take a break from the stress of constantly having to eat organic rabbit food. I instead indulge in the local cuisine, which is often tastier and healthier than what I eat at home, anyway.

I'm not trying to make you envious. I realize that many Lyme disease sufferers can't travel, but it is nonetheless beneficial for all of us to take mini-vacations from the worries of our Lyme disease lives. Watch a good movie, read a fun novel, engage in a lighthearted conversation that has nothing to do with Lyme disease, play with your dog, take up fishing. Pray for others. If you can't manage any of these things, try contemplating a flower. We need to take care of ourselves, but we also need a break from thinking and worrying about the way to health and prosperity, and not just once in awhile, but every day. It can be an effort when you don't feel well, but you may find that if and when you can manage it, it's medicine for your soul.

Forty Little Lessons of Lyme Disease

If it hadn't been for Lyme disease, I wouldn't have learned that...

1. The ability to breathe should never be taken for granted

2. Discipline is often necessary for restoration of health

3. Microwave dinners and food in a box or can aren't really food at all

4. Candy bars might be better for you than flavored yogurt

5. Cell phones, computers and hair dryers cause cellular dysfunction

6. Coffee, when served in a little red bag, can be good for you

7. Tap water isn't really safe to drink, and bottled water causes cancer

8. It's possible to swallow fifteen capsules all at once

9. Sleep is precious

10. It's not okay to lie in the grass

11. Hairspray and make-up lead to endocrine dysfunction

12. Brushing the skin with a stiff-bristled brush feels good

13. Baths and saunas are like a warm hug to the body

14. Hot cups of herbal tea are a song for the soul

15. Emotional trauma can be stored in organs besides your brain

Connie Strasheim

16. The body can heal itself more than any herb, vitamin or drug

17. Healing and forgiveness go hand in hand

18. Rushing through life causes illness and discontent

19. There is life on the other side of this world, but getting close to its door is scary

20. Loving God is easier when the mind is free of pathogens

21. The friends whom you expect to be there for you during hard times won't be, and the ones whom you don't expect, will

22. A broken heart can break the body faster than any bug

23. The immune system can be trained to kill bugs

24. You can alter your cellular behavior by speaking truth to yourself

25. God wants us to love Him for who He is, and not just His gifts

26. Living in performance mode and repressing emotions destroys the body

27. It's not what others do to you that matters but how you respond to them

28. Negativity and criticism foster biochemical dysfunction

29. Peace is in perspective, more than it is in circumstances

30. Self-sabotage is about the small things...forgetting to replace the toilet roll or denying yourself an organic steak

31. Money goes further than you think, and you don't need as much as you think

32. It's good to trust God more than science and physicians

33. Living a frenetic life of busyness starves the spirit

34. People weren't meant to thrive on false food, fast technology and superficial relationships

35. Living with mindfulness is vital for vitality

36. In weakness you can be stronger than when you truly thought you were strong

37. Your needs and wants matter to God

38. Speaking your mind in a spirit of love fosters health

39. You can't give to others until you know you are loved

40. Without the ability to love, you will never be totally healed

Chapter 16

And for a Little Humor...

Ten Reasons Why You Should Be a Professional Sofa Spud (or an Armchair Artichoke, as They Don't Move Much, Either)

1. The sofa (or chair) in your home is a comfier place to spend the day than some vinyl office chair. Plus you get a view of the living room or bedroom, instead of boring, in-your-face cubicle walls.

2. You can take as many potty breaks as you like without a boss being around to lift an eyebrow. You can even eat at your soft station.

3. You can read and write at your leisure. Whatever you want. Oprah, diet books, or a Ted Dekker novel, instead of some boring training manual, sales plan or complaint letter from a client.

Connie Strasheim

4. You can eat healthy, homemade food every day, instead of expensive, processed fast food, which your body rejects, anyway.

5. You don't have to get up at the crack of dawn, shower and then battle an hour of rush hour traffic. No, get up and make it to the sofa at your leisure. Spend the day in your jammies if you wish. And forget wasting forty-five minutes on painting your face.

6. You can have a pleasant conversation with friends, instead of spewing a stressful sales pitch to a potential customer. And forget about gossipy co-workers. You won't have to deal with that nonsense, unless you decide to turn on the television for a mid-afternoon talk show.

7. You can go to the gym and grocery store when nobody else is there. No long lines, no parking problems, no waiting to get on the Stairmaster.

8. You can work on all those quiet little hobbies you never had time for before, or all those little mental problems you've ignored for so many years. There's no busyness of a day job to distract you from your mind anymore. Trust me, this is a good thing!

9. You can talk to your furry friends (and if you don't have one, go get one, as they are pretty easy to come by) instead of listening to the whining of co-workers.

10. You can work on your goal of total health. Take advantage of it, for you may not ever have this opportunity again!

The Lyme Disease Store: Finding a Few Goofy Things to Take Home with You

Wouldn't it be great if there were an all-purpose store for Lyme disease sufferers that provided all those goods you just can't seem to find anyplace else?

Wait, there is! Now, coming to a tick town near you, it's the Lyme Disease Store, the best (and only) one-stop shop for the Lyme disease sufferer. Come purchase items for all your needs, from medication to sleepwear, or just browse if you are short on cash.

For Sale:

Eunice's Enema Bags—Strong, sturdy, and really get the garbage out, quickly, safely and effectively! On sale: two for ten dollars.

Rage Reliever—More powerful than Prozac, these specially formulated anger-management pills will help keep your relationships with your loved ones from perishing. Buy two bottles, get one free. Take the offer! After all, somebody you know probably has Lyme disease; they just don't know it yet.

Jumbo Pill Organizer—Because the ones they sell in the drugstore just aren't big enough to fit your weekly pharmacy of Lyme disease supplements.

Super-Sized Punching Bag—You thought these were only for boxers? Next time you're furious at your lot in life, have a swing at this baby! It's better than taking your misery out on your wife or husband. Hang it in your basement or garage, where there's lots of space for yelling and throwing punches.

Nature Posters—For when you can't do anything but stare at the wall, these provide you with some colorful scenes to take your mind off your life of nothingness. Caution: Not for use in those who end up envious that they can't be part of the nature scene.

Connie Strasheim

Dumb bells—For the Lyme disease sufferer, they have a much more important function than exercise. For only five bucks a dumb bell, you can rid yourself of insomnia by knocking yourself silly before bedtime. Yeah, you may have a headache by morning, but hey, at least they work better than all those sleep medications you've been taking.

Personality Disorder Bracelet—This is kind of like a medical bracelet for those with diabetes, to alert others to their ailment in a life-or-death situation. In the Lyme disease sufferer, it serves as a handy disclaimer for when others just don't understand your strange behavior.

Post-It Notes—Color-coded so you can organize your life by subject: physicians' appointments, work assignments, relationship obligations and every fragment of information that your spectacular memory cannot retain. Buy two and get one free. Post them everywhere: on the refrigerator, bathroom sink, steering wheel, nightstand, or wherever. They are as versatile as you are.

Foggy Days and Sunny Days Planner, 2008-2020—Get one of each for whatever the day may bring. Use the Foggy Days Planner when you aren't feeling stellar, as it's more compact and provides smaller squares for writing in the day's obligations. The small spaces mean you don't have to feel guilty for whatever tasks you can't fit into a Foggy Day. Choose the larger-squared Sunny Day Planner for when you are feeling better and can make up for lost time by penciling-in three times as many tasks as you did on yesterday's Foggy Day.

I-Wish-I-Had-A-Life Journal—An exceptionally great product for when life just stinks. By writing down everything that you aren't able to do, you'll have some hard core evidence for gratitude when things get better down the road.

Epsom Bubble Bath N' Salts—Who says Lyme disease sufferers should have to bathe in boring, flat, colorless salt water? Grab your rubber duckie and check these out! Enjoy sweet-scented bubbles while detoxifying with classic Epsom salts. One product, one stop, all the way!

Airline Travel Kit—Now available at the Lyme Disease Store! Yes, you are unique, dear Lyme disease sufferer. Only you would need orange earplugs and a dark eye mask to sleep whenever you aren't on an airplane. But no worries, you don't have to travel to the airport anymore for these, as the Lyme disease store now carries them for only twice the price, at ten dollars a set.

Sign-It-Yourself, All-Purpose Doctor's Letter—Set of twenty, for use on all occasions. Suggested uses: Calling in sick for work, as an excuse for not having to wait in security lines at the airport, securing pre-scriptions that your physician refuses to write for you and much more!

Emergency Snack Kit—Gluten, nut, corn, sugar and soy-free. No added hormones, pesticides, antibiotics, preservatives or other unnatural garbage. A necessity when your blood sugar plummets out in the middle of nowhere, this emergency snack kit is a nutritious lifesaver that may not have much flavor, but is faithful to get you through the day. We're not sure what's in it, but it's all good and totally organic.

Mini-Address And Phone Book—Since you've probably lost many of your friends throughout your journey with Lyme disease, we've kept this one small. Compact and lightweight, with small spaces like the Foggy Days Planner.

The Amazing Pillow-Rama Set—As a Lyme disease sufferer, you have special needs and are entitled to special treatment. While one pillow at bedtime suffices for the healthy soul, you have the honor of requiring three or four to meet your needs for slumber. We have designed the Pillow-Rama set with you in mind. Use Pillow #1 for your head, Pillow #2 to prop against your back, Pillow #3 to cuddle against your belly, and Pillow #4 as a back-up for whenever Pillows 1-3 end up on the floor from all that shish-kabobing you do during the night. What's more, our new pillow set is versatile! You can rearrange Pillows #1-4 as needed, taking all the guesswork out of which fluffy to use for each function.

Connie Strasheim

The Green Wardrobe—As a Lyme disease sufferer, you know how hard it is to make the simplest of decisions. In this wardrobe, we've removed all the guesswork from getting dressed by putting together two identical outfits, both green, which you wear every day, without having to think about what else to put on because they come with matching green underpants and green socks. Why green? Well, why not? This is a meticulously chosen color that has been scientifically proven to enable you to think about spring and warmer days ahead.

Detachable Air Purifier—For use under your clothing, this battery-operated, compact air purifier automatically releases rose-scented perfume every time your digestion malfunctions and you can't help but free that bubble building in your gut. Designed to combat even the foulest of free-floating gas.

The Little Book of Excuses—Ever wondered how to say "No" to that party invitation you already agreed to? How to decline your best friend's need for a babysitter? How to reject a date with the guy next door? This little book is chock-full of ways to let 'em down easy, with exceptionally valid excuses for the super-fatigued as a bonus.

Plastic Sympathy Doll—Blow her up and watch her shoulders expand! Designed of strong, sturdy plastic so that you can lean comfortably upon her, the Sympathy Doll provides a nice place to rest your head whenever the going gets tough. Just use your imagination a little and pretend she's a real person. That way, you won't be disappointed when she doesn't say much in response to your tears. But hey, aren't the best friends in the world the ones who simply listen?

The Lyme Dating Book—Find out whether your date is stellar marriage material by estimating his capacity to deal with pain, early nights in, a restricted diet and moments of brain fog and rage.

Pocket Lyme Dictionary, the New Transposed Word version—For when your brain can't put two and two together and you need a new, improved dictionary that makes sense only to you, the Lyme disease sufferer.

101 Things to Do on a Bad Lyme Disease Day—With everything from watching daddy longlegs move down the wall to salivating on your pillow, this compact book offers real-life suggestions from real-life Lyme disease sufferers on how to make the most (or least) of your time.

The Jerry Springer Re-Run Set—Just you can feel better about your own life.

The Temperature Chameleon—We know how a busted thyroid can mess with your body's ability to regulate your inner temperature, and that's why we've invented the Temperature Chameleon! A green turtleneck (because we really like green in this store, it reminds us of spring, and sits well with the envious feelings we have towards normal, healthy people!) that regulates the body's temperature. This new, patented fabric keeps you warm when it's warm and cold when it's cold, just like your body is supposed to do!

Spiro-Paste—Flouride-free and enhanced with cat's claw and colloidal silver for a new, healthier way to kill some bad bugs as you get ready for bed. Just squeeze a bit on your toothbrush and away you go! The spirochetes will never guess what you're up to.

Twenty Things to Do on a Date When You Both Have Lyme Disease

1.   Sit on the sofa with some chamomile tea and compare battle wounds.

     The conversation might start something like this, with Lyme Girl saying to Lyme Boy, "You know, this disease has erased my entire short-term memory. So forgive me, but I can't remember what you do for a living."

     Then Lyme Boy says to Lyme Girl, "Oh yeah, well you know what? They tell me I have Lyme rage so don't think you're the only one who suffers here!"

Connie Strasheim

2. Speaking of stimulating conversation, how about a whine and cheese party? Whoever is in symptom-flare mode can provide the whine, and the other, the cheese

3. Cuddle, pop a few benzodiazepines, put on a brain wave CD and experience sleep for the first time in a month.

4. Go for a walk and then check one another for ticks, just for the practice.

5. Stretch out on the floor and enjoy a nice cup of Colombian brew together. (Get your mind out of the gutter! I'm not talking about taking it in a red rubber bag!).

6. Have a back massage without expecting more than a two-minute session from your date due to the poop-out and pain factor. But isn't that the great thing about being on a Lyme disease date? The expectations are so low.

7. Swap supplements over dinner and discuss the latest food supply contamination problem. Don't mind the stuttering, forgetfulness and word farts of the other.

8. Have a nice dinner of spinach and spinach, with spinach for dessert, since it's the only food you both aren't allergic to.

9. Burn the midnight oil at nine and agree to another exciting night together in two weeks

10. Rent movies that don't steal adrenaline from you. That means no thriller flicks.

11. Put on some knee slappin', toe thumpin' tunes from the IRT (Immune Response Training) band, turn up the volume and watch your date's symptoms morph before your very eyes.

12. Show your date your latest Lyme rash colony and feel self-actualized when he or she says you must be doing something right in your Lyme disease regimen, since you're herxing so madly.

13. Gossip about the latest happenings on the Lyme Yahoo! Groups.

14. Get into a fight on the full moon and then kiss and make up the day after.

15. Have some Rife at your cheese and whine party and then reel together from the die-off reaction. Finally, you've found someone who really knows what you're going through.

16. Try to impress one other with knowledge about the latest and greatest Lyme disease treatments, and then suffer the effects of the Overwhelmed Factor afterwards.

17. Have a bio-energetic tapping session and discover what makes your date tick.

18. Muscle-test one another to find out whether you are really compatible. And boy, if and when your arm goes weak, run, Forrest, run!

19. Go to a sauna and sweat out toxins together. Whoever passes out first from the heat can carry the other out of the sauna.

20. Finally, discuss all the great things you'll do on your next date, knowing that there's no pressure to actually make it happen!

How a Lymie Makes a Salad: Blunders of a Lyme Body in Action

The foibles of a Lyme brain, while frustrating, can be downright laughable if you really think about them. In an attempt to channel

Connie Strasheim

irritation at my own stupidities into humor, I thought I'd share with you my typical experience of making a salad. No, really, you might relate....

I start by putzing to the refrigerator and removing a head of spinach, cucumber, cherry tomatoes and feta cheese. Then I close the fridge and open the drawer in front of me to take out a knife. Oops, wrong drawer. Well, I've only lived in this house for five months, and the kitchen does have a lot of drawers, doesn't it? I open another one and find my knife. Then open a cabinet to find a bowl to wash the vegetables in, but it seems that my mother has once again rearranged the dishes. Or has Lyme disease rearranged my brain?

I close the cabinet. Open another, and then another. Where are those bowls?

I go to the dishwasher. Aha!

I rinse the vegetables. Attempt to slice the cucumber down the middle and instead tag my thumb. Grab a paper towel but blood flows like the Nile. How can my doc be so sure that I have hypercoagulation? Sure doesn't seem like it. Manage to find a Band-Aid but decide to cut up the vegetables first, using my left hand to slice, and the side of my right hand, whose fist clutches the bloody towel and thumb, to support the cucumber. Genius. Who needs a Band-Aid, anyway? I can just walk around for the next hour, gripping a paper towel with my right hand while I use my left hand to eat. That should be an interesting challenge.

Hand taken care of, I open the refrigerator again to get the lemon juice for my dressing. Close the refrigerator and set the juice on the counter. Wait, I forgot the pesto sauce. Well, I'll just have to get it later. In the meantime, I'd better retrieve the olive oil from the pantry while I'm thinking about it.

I instead take out another knife from one of the multitudinous drawers. Now I need the pesto. I open the refrigerator, and leave it open as I scoop out pesto and dollop it on my salad. Wait, wasn't I supposed to mix the pesto with the olive oil? But I haven't even made it to the pantry yet.

Since I'm beside the refrigerator, I might as well take out the cherry-flavored Concentrace minerals to mix with my water. I leave the fridge open this time as I fill a water glass and set my salad and glass on the table.

I glance at the salad. It's still missing something. Avocado! I go to the already open fridge (I'm learning now) remove an avocado and then another knife from the knife-drawer. Cut the avocado and then wonder why I now have three dirty knives on the counter. Why should I wonder? This is Lyme brain at its best!

I remove my pharmacy of supplements from another drawer, set these beside my lunch, and make one more trek to the refrigerator to find my spirulina. Phew. I think I'm done. With only seven trips to the refrigerator, three knives and one bloody thumb, and in just ten minutes flat. Ten minutes, you say? Well, hyperactivity more than makes up for inefficiency, doesn't it?

I pick up my fork, glance at my salad and realize I forgot the oil olive. I mean, olive oil! Dang it...

Morning Malaise and the Bed Battle with the Body

How I long for those days when I used to fly out of bed at the first beeps of my alarm clock! I've never been a snooze-buttoner, but now, thanks to Lyme disease, I have to slap the sucker a half-dozen times before I am able to pull myself, kicking and screaming, out of bed.

Meanwhile, I spend the first hour of my day between the sheets, trying to convince the limbs to move. Initially, it isn't painful, because my body hasn't yet been urged to motion. Rather, twilight slumber caresses all of my parts as they linger in the softness of my pillow and mattress. I move in and out of shallow dreams, peaceful. It's only when I decide to get up that my heated debate with the body begins.

Connie Strasheim

Maybe you know what this is like. Maybe you have a similar subconscious battle with your body in the morning.

"It won't be so hard once you're up and about." I often tell my body.

"Are you sure? Sometimes you get up too early and I feel terrible for hours." It responds.

"I'm going to feel like my life is a greater waste if I lie in bed all day."

"That's your problem."

"Come on. It's been like this from day one. You've always been able to get going."

"I'm tired of this. I don't want to do it anymore. It's killing me."

"Me neither, but we have to."

"No, we don't. I would feel better just staying here. We can watch a movie in bed, later in the day."

"I want my life back. You've got to help me."

"Don't push me. You push me and I'll rebel further. Before you know it, you'll need to sleep twenty hours a day instead of ten."

"Are you threatening me? Come on, get up."

The body rolls over. "Ah, doesn't the pillow against the belly feel grand!"

"I'm sure it does. Let's go now. I've got work to do today."

"Just a few more minutes."

"For what?"

"I have to prepare for this."

"You can't prepare! You'll find all kinds of excuses to lollygag another hour."

"No, I won't." The body rolls over. "Ah yes, just a few more minutes like this. The legs love a good stretch! "

"It's ten-thirty! We should have been up at least two hours ago."

"You know the adrenal glands wouldn't have been cool with that."

"Forget the adrenals! If it were up to them, we'd be here all day!"

"I don't mind."

"Well, I do. I'm going to be really depressed if we give in to this life of nothingness. As it is, we hardly get anything done all day, anyway."

"Just a few minutes in the fetal position...maybe one more dream."

"I've had it with remembering dreams! Could you not put me into a deeper state of sleep at night, and avoid some of these absurd night-mares? They stay with me all day. I've got better things to think about."

"I can't handle this, and I'm tired of working for you. All you do is become angry with me for my efforts, anyhow."

"Of course, because you can't function like a normal, thirty-one year-old body should."

"Is that how old we are? I thought we were at least eighty."

"Get up."

"Stop telling me what to do. Listen, Miss Pushy. You need to hear me out for a minute here. Understand that all of the functions that I carry out for you require twice the effort of that of a healthy person. Asking for ten hours of sleep a night is nothing compared to what I deserve for being forced to function with cells that are flooded with creepy-crawly toxic things, the filth of industry, and the psychological garbage you fed me!"

Connie Strasheim

"The psychological garbage wasn't all my fault."

"That's it. Keep shifting the blame and I'll never work for you again."

"Do you mean to?"

"Don't you think I've tried? I can't keep up with what you ask of me. As if I was ever built to withstand so much abuse."

"Was it all that traveling around the world?"

"That was the least of it, but it helped to put us under, for sure. What fool attempts to get on a plane to go overseas for vacation or missions work five times a year, when she's already on an airplane eighteen days a month for work? Do you think I liked having to spend an additional two to four days per month trapped inside a horrible, germ-infested, pressurized metal tube? Not to mention the jet lag. I like to know what time it is. You know, rising and sleeping with the sun, that's my thing. But with you, I never knew what sun to follow."

"What about the rest?"

"I don't know, but I don't blame you for the psychological garbage. I just wish you would have paid attention to the racing heart and brain in chaos."

"I don't want to think about this. Now come on, let's go."

"What have you got to look forward to today? I'm not taking you for a walk, that's for sure."

"The adrenals are still angry about the antibiotics."

"Darn right."

"Well, I'm sorry, but they're going to have to get over it. Come on!"

The body moves. As soon as my feet hit the floor, the body rages against compliance. But we keep going, because I know that in another half-hour, it'll start to agree with me, and by evening it will be feeling so good that it won't want to go to bed—and then we'll have another battle. Often, our bodies have wisdom and it's good to listen to them. Occasionally, however, I think our conscious minds know better what we need for our health. Wouldn't you agree?

Seven Advantages to Living in Costa Rica (or Another Country!) with Lyme Disease

Being in another country can offer you unique healing advantages that you might not otherwise find at home. Below I share a few that I discovered while living in Costa Rica with Lyme disease.

1. You can be forgiven for losing track of time during a bout of brain fog, because Costa Ricans do it all the time. Heck, nobody ever shows up for meetings promptly, so now you don't have to, either.

2. You won't be frowned upon if you get your facts wrong about someone or something. People in Costa Rica don't think it's a big deal to accumulate relatively useless bits of information, such as the percentage of inhabitants who attend the theater in San Jose or the population of rats on the pacific coast.

3. Speaking of brain fog and memory, you'll be shown mercy if you happen to forget a date with another. Half the time, appointments aren't kept here, anyway.

4. People are big into alternative and natural healing remedies. They won't look at you like you're crazy when you tell them that you are treating your illness auditorily, with CD's that teach your immune system how it's supposed to behave.

5. If you are feeling fatigued and spacey, you can move at a snail's pace without locals getting impatient with you. So hand your change over to the cashier as slowly as you'd like, take your time at the restaurant, and don't worry about getting in some-

Connie Strasheim

one's way on the street (except, of course, when drivers come screaming at you full speed ahead as you cross).

6. The tropical greenery of Costa Rica brings more oxygen into the environment, which in turn scares and suffocates the tarnations out of borrelia, which thrives in an anaerobic environment.

7. Finally, most Costa Ricans still believe in and rely on God for healing and all things in life. If their beliefs rub off on you, you just might find God to be a great balm to soothe you from the loneliness of Lyme disease.

Section III

Emotional Strategies for Healing Lyme Disease

Connie Strasheim

Chapter 17

Managing Circumstantial Difficulties with the Mind

Eat Your Peas! I mean, "P's"...Those that Stand for Perseverance and Patience

Whoops. I guess I spelled that P-word wrong. I'm not actually referring to the little green veggies you used to fling at your sister from across the dinner table as a child, but that letter in the alphabet from which the words perseverance and patience are built. The two qualities we Lyme sufferers are reticent to ingest but which arm us with hope and positive energy to forge ahead with the battle of illness. Qualities that enable us to believe that we'll reach the finish line where a banner reads, "Health," just as sure as the tortoise beat the hare at his own race. Slow and steady was the motto of the turtle, and it ought to be the slogan of any Lyme disease sufferer when pursuing treat-

Connie Strasheim

ment because being a diligent slug who eats a lot of "P's" is the only way to be at peace while suffering from this illness.

This doesn't mean I know how to do it. Personally, I'm not keen on a diet of "P's." Neither am I fond of things that trudge along.

"But I want to be well now!" My body clamors instead, as I set yet another ridiculous deadline for healing from Lyme disease.

Then I wait, months and months, the deadline passes, and frustration kicks in, as it always does when I'm not well by a certain date.

Don't get me wrong; setting goals is good, but confirming a date for your health wedding can be disappointing. Especially if you are like me and believe that all dates and finish lines are subject to God's approval and re-writing.

It's astounding how often I tell myself, "I'm going to be healed of Lyme disease by this time next year, because I've been at this gerbil-in-a-wheel treatment thing for two (or three) years and that's enough! Besides, isn't two to three years the norm for recovery?"

What I'm discovering, however, is that despite the statistics, there is no certainty when it comes to healing chronic illness. Stats are just comfort food for an uncertain tomorrow, but that's where the "P's" come to the rescue. Nobody wants to digest perseverance and patience, because it's so much effort, but the sooner we strive to incorporate them into our diet, the more sanity and strength we'll have during recovery, in a journey fraught with maybe's.

Indeed, without them, we would be left disgruntled and in despair by circumstances that shuffle us along a path of too many twists, turns and disappointing dead ends.

Remembering that Your Brain Still Works on "Stupid" Days

Do you recall that old Sesame Street song you used to hear as a kid? It started out like this..."Sunny days, sweeping the, clouds away.... And then the music, "Dee dum dum...." Well, one day I had a new version of that tune playing through my mind. It went..."Foggy days, bringing the, clouds to stay...." And then my music, "Dumb dumb dumb...."

Can I vent for just a moment? I mean, you might feel better knowing you're not the only foggy freak on the planet.

It never fails to astound me what an utter mess Lyme disease can make of my neurons. While the effects of borrelia upon the brain bring about devastating symptoms, such as depression and forgetfulness, today I have a different bone to pick with the bacteria. It has to do with the organism switching my thought processes over to slithering slug speed. Whenever this happens, I want to throw my computer out the window and forget attempting to put any of my garbled-up thoughts into words. Can you relate?

Yeah, consider that it just took me nearly an hour to crank out four measly paragraphs for this book. Besides the sheer block of not knowing what to say or how to say it, I kept hitting the "delete" key to fix transposed words, agreement errors and ridiculous redundancies. That's the tortoise brain in action! Woo hoo, turn it on and watch it go! Okay, so spending an hour on four simple paragraphs wouldn't be so bad for someone who doesn't write often, but I do it every day! (It's okay, put the violin away.)

Ah, but I can only complain so much. Kicking and screaming, I grudgingly admit that on some days, I have return glimpses of times when I could run like a hare and think like the clearest blue sky (okay, so a sky with a few clouds), and not only in writing, but in all things. Days where tasking felt efficient, and the hours and production mill ran like clockwork.

Connie Strasheim

It's good for all of us to reminisce and be thankful for those times, especially when we have a foggy snail-slug-tortoise you-name-the-animal frustrating day. Doing so will remind us that we still have amazing brains that work, even if sometimes Lyme disease tries to convince us otherwise, and help us to appreciate and take advantage of the good days when the mind goes and flows as God intended. Or, to have gratitude for its ability to function at all! Considering that our brains are forced to contend with the filth of a billion bugs, if you are able to read this book, I'd say you are doing pretty well! I mean, it could be worse, couldn't it?

Pay Attention to the Small Changes When You're Fed Up with Your Regimen

Why are you complaining? Just because you have a few dozen Lyme disease therapies you're supposed to do every day! Everyone has a daily regimen, and you should consider yourself fortunate. Why? Because yours probably isn't as strictly regulated as the more productive human who has to get up at the same hour every day, drive to the same job and complete the same tasks until it's time to go home and hit the haystack.

Yes, I know, being busy all day long with therapy "have-to's" is wearing. While your friends assume that you must be bored off your heels because you aren't working an 8-5 job outside the home, saying, "Well, what DO you do with your time?" truth is, you don't have any free time!

For starters, your inconsistent sleep routine messes everything up. You might only have twelve or fourteen semi-productive sluggish hours in the day, since you toss and turn in twilight slumber during the other ten hours. And since your brain and body don't function well, it takes you longer than the average human to get things accomplished. So between yoga, ozone insufflations, body brushing, prayer and visualization therapy, Epsom salt baths, enemas, fixing nutritious meals, Rifing, doctor appointments, saunas, on-line shopping for supplements, research and all the time that it takes to mix n' match and gobble up those supplements, your hours are filled.

On days when your symptoms flare and improvement feels like an illusion, you especially resent pouring thousands of hours and dollars into treatments and caring for your body. Why should you bother, when you are just rewarded with more pain, fatigue and fog?

On such days, you must remind yourself that little changes count and that progress cannot be measured by how bad you feel when you're having a down day, but by how good you feel on your better days. Days when the brain fog and fatigue retreat for awhile and the shackles of pain become loosened. Recall those days when you are fed up with your six million supplements, hours on the Rife machine and visits to the doctor. Think about how, on such days, the sunshine feels a bit warmer upon your face and how, with the passage of time, the colors of life seem to be getting brighter. Notice how your energy is slowly increasing, with each good day that you have, and acknowledge that your regimen is working, even if just a little.

If you don't seem to be making progress, however, realize that it still wouldn't be in your best interest to abandon your regimen, because you might be worse off without it, and you want to keep doing whatever is necessary to get your health back. Anyway, if you were completely healthy, you'd still have a regimen. Your responsibilities would simply be different.

Grieving Over a Life Lost and the Humdrum of Existence

Boy, has this Lyme disease been a shock to my lifestyle. Can you relate? In twenty-four hours flat, I went from a life of ultra-stimulation to couch tater humdrum. As I think of my friends, out mountain biking on this gorgeous spring day, I sit on the sofa in my dark basement and do what I do every day of my now quiet existence: read, write or perform Lyme disease treatments. Not that I don't enjoy

Connie Strasheim

these things, but a little recreation and social life, along with some meaningful work, would be nice from time to time, too.

Today I don't feel like pacifying my disquietude by musing over the higher good that stillness and illness are supposed to bring. I said my prayers this morning. I see the blessing of having more time to spend with God, but I can't help but feel that this sort of lifestyle should be reserved for those who are in their last days of life, not for a lady who should be in the prime of her existence.

Can you empathize with my inability to be strong all of the time? Is there any room for grieving the life we have lost? If so, how can we do that and still accept what is?

Sometimes I think I can win against God's design for my life by rebelling against this illness and refusing to find peace in it. Like a child who holds her breath until she turns blue because Daddy won't give her a lolly, I think that I can somehow punish my creator by refusing to accept this stinking Lyme lot. Of course, in the end, it hurts only me and gets me no further along the healing path.

Not that God wants me to be sick. In fact, He may want me healed in the fastest manner possible, but why do I have this dark premonition that doing so requires me to first be okay with things as they are? Do I fear that embracing a life void of recreation will resign me to it?

The battle rages on. You may notice that my blurbs on Lyme disease are paradoxical. I'm not a hypocrite but my thoughts are divided by the whims of my biochemistry, my broken nature and my relationship with God. On some days, my mind is in a beneficial place, but on others, I lollygag in the tar pit because it's nice and cool there, and the higher road just feels too high.

I guess I could find a nice book and sit out in the sunshine. It would be some kind of compromise that would help me put the self-inflicted Merlot and Munster party to rest, as it dresses up the monotony of a routine that seldom changes.

If you are like me, you feel fortunate to have had the ability to do so much before you became ill, but it has been painful to lose that life. So maybe, just for one day, week, month or year, it's okay to be sad for what you've lost. Grieving is part of the healing process, and you have a right to your despondency, as you learn to accept the new life that Lyme disease has given you. Ironically, it is the grieving process that might bring you to an acceptance of your circumstances, which in turn may lead you towards a better life than the one that you lost.

"Will I EVER Get Better?"...Hope for When You Crash

You know the scenario. You start a therapy that improves your symptoms. You fly high and feel good for a few days, weeks, or even months, before...SPLAT! You crash like a bird shot with a BB gun. Your wings are broken. You forget about freedom. The same ol' symptoms have returned to engulf you with fatigue and fog that are fiercer than ever.

You're furious at your broken body for betraying you. "What's wrong with you that nothing ever seems to work? Isn't (fill in the blank here) years of this illness enough? Couldn't you one day just function normally—and stay that way?"

Or maybe you get mad at God, or your spouse or your dog. Or your pillow. Just something. You've been trying so hard. You've been spending so much money and effort and life's hours only to have Big, Bad Borrelia triumph over your not-so-spiffy tactics. You are fed up. I know. I am, too. Often.

The ebb and flow of symptoms also causes your brain to become subject to warped interpretations of healing. This isn't news to you either, but it's funny how, no matter how often you tell yourself this, you still fall into a tar pit of despair on days when symptoms drag you down with their iron chains.

Connie Strasheim

"I'm never going to get better!" A voice screams inside of you. But after awhile, the clouds part, your symptoms abate and suddenly the world looks rosy again, and of course you are going to heal! How could you have ever believed that you wouldn't?

It's worse when you feel good for a longer period of time, say, several months, because then your hopes soar even higher, before BOOM! You crash again. But this time, your arse hurts more because you've managed for a time to get above the clouds.

Still, you pick yourself back up and dare to hope a little, because life leaves you no choice but to do this or stay flat on your face, inhaling sludge.

And after awhile, you start to feel good again, and as you dare to spread your wings, the process starts all over again.

Maybe one day, you won't fall from such heights. Or you'll at least reap some kind of reward for your amazing perseverance. In the meantime, take joy in a rump that becomes more bruised with every crash landing, because it means that you are reaching greater heights each time. That means progress. Take joy especially in the great disappointment that follows. It means you had reason to hope in the first place. And that hope will rise again.

Focusing on Nine Lessons of Chronic Illness

We should never cease to see the sterling in the storm cloud, and that includes the great lessons that illness can bless us with. Some of these may include:

1. Learning how to slow down, because there is no way you would have stopped your breakneck pace of life if it weren't for Lyme disease. You realize that life is about being, as much as it is about doing.

2. Realizing that it's vital to give the body nutrition, not garbage. The healthy and sick alike know this, but being sick, you learn that there's more to it than just eating a few greens, and the difference between depression and peace of mind, between being bedridden or functional, is often in what you eat.

3. Obtaining the knowledge that our food supply and environment are heavily contaminated. By being aware of this on a deep level, you can make well-informed choices for your habits and lifestyle.

4. Learning that your worth isn't in your ability to be productive. You can be couch-bound and still have purpose in life. While it may be the most difficult lesson to learn, joy is not found as much in the external factors of life as the internal.

5. Developing compassion towards others. Yes, you now know what it's like to be disabled and poor, and your heart goes out without judgment to the ill, handicapped, homeless and forsaken.

6. Learning to focus on God and developing a spiritual life as your reason for being. You might not have acknowledged God otherwise. You would not have understood that true peace comes from developing a relationship with your creator.

7. Learning to cultivate new talents and hobbies. You can't often get out of bed, and your brain is like a lava lamp, globbing every which way, but the neurons still plod along, and your limbs still function. You've learned how to make jewelry, and it's more fun than you imagined. Maybe you'll take up watercolor painting next.

8. Becoming a health connoisseur and teaching friends and family what you know. You've never had a passion for healing others before Lyme disease, but you suddenly find it intriguing. Maybe you can better help them now to find solutions to their own ailments.

Connie Strasheim

9. Learning that you can get by with less financially than you thought. That your dollars or pesos stretch further than you would have believed and that despite not being able to splurge for luxury items anymore, your basic needs are still being provided for, and you don't really need a new camera to be happy.

The Fun House Monster...Hope for When You're on a Wild Mental Ride

The Fun House Monster moved into my brain about twenty years ago, right along with borrelia burgdorferi. It came to distort my thoughts and used to stand me in front of its favorite fun-house mirror, where I would see a warped view of myself, others and life's circumstances.

The Fun House Monster shouted "Boo!" at every turn, leaving me paranoid over events that for healthier folks would have carried little or no emotional charge. It took me on wild rides of irrationality and rage and enticed me to believe that others were out to get me. It put me on a merry-go-round of emotions, up and down, until I became sick to my stomach. Another one of its favorite pastimes was luring me onto its roller coaster and pressing the fast forward button, where the soaring and plummeting of my spirits would become so intense that I thought my brain would fall out of my body and my body out of my brain.

Fortunately, as I have treated my Lyme disease, the Fun House Monster has become less influential in its ability to take me for rides. As I have detoxified my body, as I have dealt with the phantoms of my past, my reason has grown more powerful, my emotions more stable, and, as a result, the monster hasn't been able to drag me in front of its fun-house mirrors as often as it used to. It can't coax me onto the roller coaster, and the nauseating merry-go-round visits are becoming infrequent. As I heal and spend less time in the fun park that isn't so much fun, I'm able to replace the monster's fun house mirror with my own mirror of truth, which doesn't distort and twist events and my relationships with others in a bizarre, ridiculous way. Instead, it presents a more rational, kind world, with people who are more loveable and a god who is more loving. And the longer I'm able to keep the Fun House Monster at bay, the more I see the world as I believe my creator intended for me to see it.

If, on some days you feel you've entered the Loony Toons theme park with a Fun House Monster for your guide, take heart; your mind can heal as you treat your Lyme disease, and the beast will one day leave your brain, for good.

Connie Strasheim

Chapter 18

Harnessing the Power of Belief, Thought and Words

Get Healthy by Getting out of Victim Mode

"Poor me!"

Yes, it's time to eat some worms. You're broke, jobless, and you have nobody with whom to cuddle at night because you're too sick to be in a romantic relationship. Nope, you seem to have no purpose in life except to exist like a mushroom in the ground, hoping that whoever stops by doesn't end up squashing you, as you spend your days feeling like the Tar Pit Baby bulldozer has run over your brain and body. Yes, you truly have a right to an orchestra of a thousand violins at your next pity party.

Thank God for pity parties! What would you do without two dozen other Lyme disease sufferers to whip out their own little stringed instruments of sympathy and play a daily concerto for you on the Internet Yahoo! support groups? How would you survive without

Connie Strasheim

those at church, who lay hands on you every week and pray for your healing? What would you do without your barf bag buddies who are always there to receive your innards whenever you need to telephone them to let it all out?

At least you aren't alone, and thank goodness that the government and your Aunt Charity are helping you with your living expenses, since you are so feeble and frail and can't make it on your own.

What would you do without your warm blankie of self-righteousness? Boy, doesn't it feel good? You can wrap it ever more tightly about you every time a friend of yours gets married, gets a promotion or otherwise experiences some stroke of good fortune that you, of course, know you'll never get because you have Lyme disease, and that means a life of disaster.

Yet, you concede a bit of thanks to God for the small donations of your friends and family, who enable your survival on Scary Planet Earth.

I now give you the right to smack me for my apparent condescension. Just as long as you know that I need the concerto and intoxicating red wine, too, as well as the charity of others. Also, I *do* believe that God intended for us to bear one another's burdens and that it's okay to need a Linus blanket or a shoulder or an ear.

But here's the thing. If we aren't careful, illness does this deceptive thing with the charity we receive and our difficult position as Lyme disease sufferers.

My dear Lymefolk, it takes charity and dependency and turns us into victims.

By encouraging us to depend upon others, it quietly sends us the message that we aren't capable of taking care of ourselves. But just because we can't work doesn't mean that we are helpless human beings, does it?

By calling ourselves disabled, it urges us to assume a victimizing new identity that precludes us from finding health. But in some ways, haven't we been re-enabled?

By allowing us to complain to others, we are given a license to not take responsibility for our hardship. It's easier to complain and solicit compassion than it is to find the good in the day and work towards healing. But wallowing is disempowering, isn't it?

By reiterating our difficulties, the idea of "Poor Me" continues to thrive in our minds and bodies. But we can't heal without first killing the ol' PM, something a victim would never dare to do!

By blaming our parents, our spouse or our Uncle Hothead for our illness, we've handed the government of our bodies over to them for their tyrannical rule, but they aren't responsible for who we are today. Only we are.

The greatest lie in the world is that others make us angry, sad or sick. If we truly assumed power over our lives and well-being, we would know that it is how we respond to the Uncle Hothead's of the world that determines whether we are victors or victims.

It's easy to fall into the victim trap. Because Lyme disease requires us to rely heavily upon others, we can easily be misled into thinking that our destiny hinges upon someone else's charity towards us. We must decide that handing over the power of our lives and happiness to other people or circumstances is counter-productive to healing.

Often, we can't control what happens to us, but we can control, at least to some degree, our minds, which is what ultimately crowns us Victor or Victim. So will you be a Poor Disabled Lymie, or a healthy soul with some physical symptoms? You decide.

Connie Strasheim

Telling Your Truth to the World...Your Health May Depend Upon It

Did you know that much of illness results not from physical toxins or infections, but from a lack of healthy boundaries in relationships? (For more information on boundaries, have a look at Dr. Cloud's and Dr. Townsend's book series on the subject: (www.cloudtownsend.com). Contrary to what you might think, boundaries aren't bad. They aren't about putting up walls between you and your loved ones, but rather, establishing communication patterns in a way that gets your needs, as well as the needs of your loved ones, met in a healthy way.

If you don't have healthy boundaries, you'll be suppressed in your ability to communicate your beliefs, thoughts, needs and wants— basically, your inner truth, to yourself and others. The result is conflict between you and the world, because what you hold on the inside doesn't match what is expressed on the outside, verbally or with actions. As a consequence, your body suffers under the burden of the lie, or the inconsistency that exists between your belief, thought or need, and your behavior.

The old adage, "be true to yourself" has great merit. Living out of sync with who you are can wreak an earthquake of havoc on your internal world. In fact, some mental healthcare practitioners believe that most people who suffer from chronic illness have a history of serious boundary problems.

The founders of Quantum Techniques, Stephen and Beth Daniel, (www.quantumtechniques.com), in their Quantum Techniques Client Manual, write that your inner truth will be communicated to the world, in one form or another. If it isn't appropriately expressed through your behavior and modes of communication, then the body will take charge and clamor to be heard through physical symptoms.

If, for example, others ask things of you that you can't give, and you don't know how to say "no" to these requests for fear of rejection or some other motive, your body may say "no" for you. How does it do this? By coming down with a bout of the flu or manifesting some other symptom so that you literally can't perform what has been asked of you. As bizarre as it may seem, your body is trying to protect you and do for you what you will not do for yourself.

Bottom line? Without a healthy ability to express yourself, and especially to communicate your needs to others, your immune system will struggle mightily to help you recover from Lyme disease.

Don't despair. None of us lives totally in accord with our inner truth. We silence ourselves because we don't want to hurt other people's feelings. We don't say what we know to be right because we fear rejection, even though it may mean we will suffer more in the long haul for it. We haven't learned to believe in our heart of hearts that loving others means being honest with them, instead of pleasing them, by showing or telling them what we think they want to hear.

Breaking unhealthy boundary patterns can help you to heal on a deeper level as you let go of the need for approval, knowing that you are worthy and loveable no matter how others react to you and that your value doesn't depend on their opinions of you.

Setting boundaries implies a willingness to risk self-expression in the name of healing. Not only will you love yourself more for doing it, but others will love you more for your honesty, too. What follows is not only a healing of your soul and spirit, but also your body.

Vanquishing Fear: the Sneaky, Slow Killer

To varying degrees, we all operate out of both fear and love. Living in love may be the greatest determinant of health, while fear opens the door to illness and keeps us on our sickbeds. Fear often works its pernicious magic upon us in subtle ways, so that we disregard its mechanisms. And perhaps the danger to the immune system isn't found as much in the huge cascades of tears or in the fireworks displays of rage as it is in the barely discernable tremors of the soul caused by fear. Learning to recognize and remove the triggers for fear can help us to dig ourselves out of the ditch of chronic illness.

Connie Strasheim

Fear is wily, often subtle, quiet and yet powerful. It hides in the little irritations; in the way we offer plastic smiles to Uncle Joe and in the way we rush through our breakfast in order to make it to work on time. It is found whenever we check our watches every fifteen minutes to make sure we're still on schedule. It rises up while driving, when we nearly miss the exit, and it makes an appearance when we show up at a party, wondering if we'll impress in our seam-splitting dress. It vocalizes itself in the sighs and snippy remarks of the day; it causes us to furrow our brows when we look at our bank accounts, and to bite our nails whenever a new Lyme symptom pops up from out of nowhere.

Fear thrives on secrets, suppression and manipulation. It teaches us that it's not okay to say "no" to others; it admonishes us to hide our sadness and pain, and it drives us to attend church when we don't really believe in God. It compels us to desperately search for answers to the question of illness, as we spend thousands of dollars on supplements.

It wears a multitude of faces and is a master of disguise, tricking its servant into believing that pride, shame, guilt and the need for approval aren't really manifestations of its mighty personality. However it operates, if fear maintains a persistent, pervasive presence in the chronic Lyme disease sufferer, biological processes become skewed and the person will have a more difficult time recovering from illness.

Unfortunately, Lyme disease causes neurological dysfunction, financial and other hardships that make it difficult for us to kick fear from our minds. Yet by laboring to do so, through prayer, meditation, affirmations of love and therapies that reach the subconscious mind, as well as a conscious decision to slow down and live mindfully, as we surrender our lives to our creator and to circumstances, we can reduce fear's influence in our lives.

Following are some specific strategies that can be helpful for healing physiological and trauma-based reasons for fear:

Binaural Beat Therapy

This process slows brain wave patterns through a CD of sounds that have the effect of pushing the mind towards higher levels of reorganization. In its reorganization, the brain adopts a higher tolerance to negative stimuli. Positive emotional changes, including a greater tolerance to stress and the elimination of pervasive fear, are some of its benefits. For more information on this technique and where to purchase CD's, visit: www.centerpointe.com.

EFT-Emotional Freedom Technique

This is a technique that you can do at home and which has tremendous healing benefits if done on a daily basis. By tapping with the fingertips on the body's meridians, or energy channels, as you repeat affirmations, harmful thinking patterns can be eliminated from the mind. The effects of this strategy can often be felt in weeks. Information on how to perform the technique can be found at: www.emofree.com.

NET- Neuro-Emotional Technique

Negative experiences are not just stored in the conscious part of our minds, but in our bodies, as well. The nervous system, in particular, carries memories of the past and is conditioned to respond in a certain way to stimuli, based on our history. As discussed later in this book, NET is a healing procedure involving touch and manipulation of the body's bio-meridians in order to de-condition the autonomic nervous system so that it responds differently to stimuli. More information can be found at: www.netmindbody.com.

Anxiety and Phobia Workbook

This is a wonderfully comprehensive book on how to treat anxiety disorders, fear and phobias. It includes information on the causes, prevention and treatment of these, and includes information for emotional healing on a holistic level, incorporating diet, lifestyle, and other factors into its approach. You can find this book on the Internet at: www.amazon.com.

Connie Strasheim

Is Your Subconscious Keeping You Sick?...Discovering the Truth Behind Blocks to Healing

Don't let the title of this section fool you into thinking that I'm blaming you for your illness. Self-flagellation is never productive for healing, and besides, why on God's green planet would anyone choose to be sick? Isn't it bad enough that physicians tell us that our illness is all in our heads? Yet while on a conscious level most people don't choose to be ill, sometimes the quiet motivations of the subconscious mind refute our conscious desires. These are worth addressing, since our bodies are influenced by the mind's agenda.

Unrecognized or unacknowledged beliefs like, "I don't deserve to heal" or, "The only way I'll be loved by my family is if I am sick," are some of these and can keep us in the Lyme disease Inferno.

Additionally, the subconscious may be using symptoms as a means of providing you with secondary gains from your illness or getting needs met that you refuse to get met on a conscious level. These may include: feeling safe at home where you won't be criticized by a boss; receiving comfort from not having to figure out what to do with your life; obtaining sympathy or attention from family members, and taking pleasure in your camaraderie with fellow Lyme disease sufferers. Or maybe you need to feel useful to other sick people and being sick yourself is the only way to accomplish that. The possibilities are endless.

Discovering the hidden motivations behind illness can be difficult and may require the assistance of a therapist, but they are important to identify because they factor into some people's recovery from Lyme disease. By healing underlying wounds, challenging lie-based belief systems and understanding on a deep level that we can get all of our needs met without the use of symptoms, we will be enabled to recover more fully.

How Words Alter Your Physical Reality

"Sticks and stones may break my bones, but words will never hurt me."

Whoever wrote that must have been in serious denial. Poor guy. We all know words can hurt, and heal, in more ways than one. Have you ever wondered if words can heal you of Lyme disease?

It has been scientifically proven that thinking, writing and speaking words of healing can alter a person's health, but there's more to it than just positive thinking.

Experiments have been done in which specific thoughts have been directed towards plants, people and bacteria, with the result that these organisms become biologically altered to conform to the thoughts that have been sent to them. This can happen even if the object isn't present in the same room with the person practicing the thought. Such experiments have also been performed using written and spoken words, with similar results.

This evidence is scientific, but it spills over into the realm of faith, too. In the book of proverbs in the Bible, for instance, it is written in verse 18:21 that, "death and life are in the power of the tongue," and, "the tongue of the wise is health" (verse 12:18). Judging by these verses, it would seem that we choose to be sick or healthy, depending upon the words we speak.

While prayer and positive affirmations may be the most obvious ways in which you can use words to effectuate healing, consider that every word you think, speak and read brings about tangible, observable consequences. If we can affect plants with our thinking, how much more can we alter the state of our health with our mind!

In general, do words of optimism and light proceed from your mouth, or do you curse the highway, your mother and the potato you're peeling for dinner? Do you proclaim to others how horrible you feel, or do you begin the day with an optimistic declaration that you are

Connie Strasheim

healing more and more each day (even if you don't feel like it!)? If you awaken in the morning with a lament over your aching limbs, are you able to replace it with praise that you can still walk, talk or see?

Take heed of your inner monologue and outer dialogue. In doing so, you may discover that the words that you say to yourself and others can powerfully affect your healing.

Creating an Alphabet Soup of Abundance in Your Life

You never get a break, do you? Yeah, me neither. I don't have the picket fence, two dogs and 2.5 kids, with a perfect husband and cool career. It doesn't mean the heavens are dumping on me, though at times I'm tempted to think so.

Whoever decided that the American dream was necessary for happiness, anyway? I wonder if there's some unwritten rule that unless you have: A) the dog, B) the great job, C) the loving hubby (or wife!) with a few kids to boot, D) the big house, and E) perfect health, then F), your life is a failure! If whether we decided to wake up and smile in the morning depended upon us meeting all of these criteria, then many of us Lyme disease sufferers would be looking mighty sad!

Okay, so life is easier when you get to eat some good alphabet soup, but maybe it's time to re-write the alphabet and start seeing your life from a place of prosperity and abundance instead of from a place of scarcity. Get rid of that F word, because your life is not a failure!

As challenging and laughable as it may seem at times, it's important to believe that you have all that you need, right now, for your happiness. It may mean speaking aloud an acknowledgment to God that you believe that all your needs are being met in the best manner possible right now, even if you don't entirely believe it, and enumerating those things that you are glad about in your life. The simple stuff, such as your bed in the homeless shelter and the rice you get to eat for dinner. But go further and have a smile at your crème de anise toothpaste, your flannel jammies and your new Lyme disease herb. Praise your Colombian decaf, the fact that you have at least one friend to speak to on the phone, and a few movies to watch when you are too sick to do anything else.

Even better, attempt to see your pain and suffering from a place of plenteousness. What you are going through (please humor me and hold the tomatoes) is a unique experience that will teach you a multitude of lessons if you allow it to. Be happy that you don't have to battle traffic in the morning on the way to a job that you hate, and that you now have time to take care of all those little dark demons that you've ignored for so many years.

Keep going; there's more good stuff if you choose to see it. So create your own alphabet soup of abundance, instead of allowing it to be defined by society's standards.

Countering Despairing Thoughts with Affirmations

You know the deal. Some days you awaken and manage to praise God or your dog for a decent night's rest (which means five solid hours without turning circles like a kabob over a spit). Other days, you wake up, feeling like a cartoon character whose body has been plugged into an electrical socket, run over by the Black Mack truck, and then flung over a cliff. On those days, if you are like me, you open your eyes and curse the day.

'THIS LIFE SUCKS!' You scream inside, or maybe even aloud, then begin a chain of laments, which seals the deal on a day that's destined to be a bummer.

It's understandable and justifiable to feel sorry for yourself, but, sadly, it compounds the problem of illness and pulls you another step away from your goal of health.

Connie Strasheim

Unfortunately and fortunately, the mind matters, even though speaking positive words of health to the body when every one of your parts is throbbing or sobbing often feels like walking along a precipice of impossibility.

But you just have to. If you want to get out of this fix, you must stop the daily Song of Laments.

I'm not saying that it's not okay to grieve. Grieving is necessary, and watering a few plants with your tears is good and healthy. Just don't do it every day if you can help it. Plants don't need that much water.

Here's the strategy. As the negative thoughts begin to tumble from your mind, first thing in the morning, grab onto them and refute them, one after the other, before they escape from you like wild horses destined for a bitter horizon.

Whenever I do this, it feels like a battle between two alter egos: Hissy Fit and the Brain Police. My typical "silent" conversations go something like this:

Hissy Fit: Ugh. Can't I awaken just ONE day without back pain?

The Brain Police: Stop it right there!

Hissy Fit: What a waste of a life. I'll bet my 93 year-old Grandma doesn't feel this bad.

The Brain Police: Would you like to spend the day in a mental prison?

Hissy Fit: This is the truth of how I feel!

The Brain Police: It doesn't matter. You must tell yourself that you are being healed, more and more each day.

Hissy Fit: How can I say this? It's not manifesting in my body!

The Brain Police: Well, your other option is the mental prison. You can't heal as long as you mope and moan over all that's wrong with you.

Hissy Fit: (Gritting her teeth). Okay. Well, uh, then...Thank you, God, for this day...I'm really grateful that I can get out of bed...Thank you for this box-spring mattress...For my eyesight...Wait, I don't believe any of this! Dang it, my neck aches. Why must I awaken every morning with so much heaviness in my chest?

The Brain Police: Don't make me lock you up!

Hissy Fit: Uh...I speak healing to this body. I know you are healing me, God...er, more and more...I know this won't last forever....

The Brain Police: That's it! Just hang in there another hour with those thoughts, and by the time you get out of bed, you'll find yourself able to believe a little differently. Remember, though, you're on probation, and tomorrow we'll have to talk again.

Hissy Fit: I'll never get out of this prison!

The Brain Police: Don't start with me!

Hissy Fit: I'm sorry. I can't help it.

The Brain Police: Yes, you can! And if you keep up the mental exercises, it will become progressively easier for you to get out of this dark place. Just continue to obey the rules for inner peace, and one day, you'll be set free.

Your battle may not be with an alter ego, or you may not recognize it as such. The important thing is that you take heed of your destructive thoughts and create affirmations to refute them whenever they bombard you in moments of pain or weakness. The rebuttals will literally help to re-wire your mind, which will, in turn, aid in the healing of your body.

Connie Strasheim

"But I Deserve to Be Well!"...How a Spirit of Entitlement Fosters Misery and How to Overcome It

Do you think that the world, or God, should give you your health back? Have you ever been tempted to think that because you've done good things for others or because you have had a tragic life that you now deserve to be healthy and happy? Do you think that if God really loved you, He'd make your life cozy and give you health, wealth and prosperous relationships?

Yes, even Job, one of the Godliest characters in the Bible, remained perplexed by the fact that God took away his health, family and wealth, when he had faithfully served Him for many years.

In my travels to over forty-five nations, I've often noticed that it's the impoverished, sick and those stricken by the worst hardships who have the most gratitude for their lives. In the poorest of countries, these people aren't fed or clothed properly, can't make use of their talents for lack of resources, their children often don't reach adulthood and their destiny is to die from hunger, disease or war. I used to wonder how it was possible that they weren't angry with God, because their lives were filled with such tragedy.

Yet many of them expressed gratitude for their mere existence. They didn't believe that their maker owed them anything, and they were thankful for every grain of rice that was given to them. Many placed their hope in an afterlife, in the promise of a "happily eternity ever after" because it enabled them to endure—and that hope was sufficient for them.

I have since realized that part of the problem with my questioning is that it reflects my worldview of what it means to be provided for, as well as a false belief that gratitude is a function of circumstance. While I now know that it is not, incorporating that truth into my heart has been difficult.

As Lyme disease sufferers, it's only human to be furious at our maker for allowing us to live a life dominated by inactivity and pain, but it can be a problem if we allow this attitude to remain constant. Ingratitude and wondering "Why me?", however unfair circumstances are, poison the body, foster unhappiness and can hinder our healing unless we get past them.

If anxiety and depression rank high on your Lyme disease symptom list, changing your thoughts can be difficult. If society, friends and family members have helped to ingrain into your psyche the idea that life owes you health, happiness and the attainment of material wealth, then vanquishing it may require tremendous discipline.

Don't think I'm telling you that you deserve to be in the mess of Lyme disease. Believing that you are worthy of health and life's comforts isn't the same as demanding them from your creator or from life, or feeling that you are entitled to them.

A good place to start healing is by praying and meditating upon your thoughts and consciously seeking to change those that smack of a spirit of entitlement. Consciously thanking God and focusing on what you have been given, instead of what you have not, is especially profitable. It may include saying "thank you" for tragedy, but notice how your heart and mental state are changed by two degrees every time you make a conscious decision to do so. Gratitude is a discipline, but one worth pursuing so that you can banish the counter-productive spirit of entitlement that keeps you rooted in illness.

"Why Me?"...Don't Even Ask the Question

Well, why not you? Yes, it is a cruel and crude answer to the question of suffering, but you gotta admit that asking "Why me?" isn't going to bring you any profitable answers, either.

Don't flagellate yourself, thinking that God or life is out to punish you and that you deserve to have Lyme disease. Forget the lie that this was

Connie Strasheim

supposed to happen to you and that you can somehow change life's rules about fairness.

Instead of comparing yourself to your wealthy, healthy neighbor, and asking, "Why me?" mentally jump on a plane to Rwanda, have a look at the sick children there and perhaps you won't feel as though you've been singled out for such agony. While weddings and holidays are spectacular occasions for noticing how much better off friends and family are than you, if you must stop attending social events in order to feel better about your lot in life, then please do so! At least counter the envy with a visit to the BBC newspage, where you'll see that it isn't only you who has been served a hefty handful of hardship.

Your pain is valid, but asking the question, "Why me?" creates a martyrdom that puts you in the victim seat and keeps you from moving forward. Even if you knew the answer to the question of why the apparently evil have good health while nice folks like you suffer, what good would it do for you to have that answer? It wouldn't get you any further along in your healing journey.

Allow yourself to be okay with being chosen by life for this trial. It doesn't mean that you have to resign yourself to it or love being there; it simply means that you accept that life is unfair and can be tragic. Embrace the idea that greater good can come from your experience with Lyme disease than if you'd been left to make of your life the perfect kingdom of circumstance that you think it should be. And then stop asking, "Why, me?", as you move onward in your healing journey.

Sub-personalities of the Anxious Lyme Disease Sufferer...Combating the Critic, Victim, Perfectionist and Worrier

I have to finish this article today. Oh dear, what if I can't? Shoot, I'm running out of time! Figures—I can never seem to manage my life. Then again, it's society's fault I feel so pressured to perform!

What's wrong with this conversation? In just two and a half lines, I've made myself into a perfectionist, worrier, critic and victim, the four sub-personalities found in people suffering from anxiety disorders, according to E. J. Bourne, author of *The Anxiety and Phobia Workbook*. These personalities can also be found in Lyme disease sufferers who suffer symptoms of anxiety.

If anxiety ails you, you are likely to have some combination of all four of these sub-personalities, and perhaps one or two that stand out in your behavioral and/or thinking patterns. The one thing these personalities all have in common is that they are based on fear and lies and have little, if anything, to do with reality.

Circumstances of hardship that Lyme disease sufferers endure help create these dysfunctional sub-personalities, but you can learn to spot them whenever they slither into your thoughts, so that you can eventually get rid of them, for good.

Let's begin with the perfectionist. It's that little personality which tells you that you're always falling short of your goals and that you need to push harder and perform better. It thrives on the word "should" and tries to convince you that your self-worth is dependent upon externals, such as job performance, acceptance by others, and your ability to give and receive love. Its expectations are sky-high, and it constantly raises the bar on achievement. Its end goal is to promote chronic stress and burnout.

Then the personality of the critic comes along to tell you how short you've fallen of your perfectionist goals. It reminds you of how you can never do anything right, and it's good at initiating beat-up sessions with your psyche. It constantly compares you with others, and convinces you that they are somehow better than you. It never allows you to make a mistake, is the initiator of all put-downs and name-calling, and is a pro at promoting low self-esteem as it exalts your weaknesses and inadequacies, whether these are real or imagined.

Then there's the worrier, whose favorite phrase is, "What if?" It throws you propositions, such as, "What if you can't achieve your goals? What if you can't let go of being critical of yourself? What if you stay sick forever? What if you suffer anxiety for the rest of your life?" It loves to create worst case scenarios and overestimates the odds of bad things happening. It also conjures up images of potential failure or catastrophe and is a real trophy winner in the game of anxiety promotion.

Finally, the victim speaks in a cozy, self-righteous voice by assuring you that it's not your fault that you are a critical, worrying perfectionist. Or that you can't help being a psychological mess and that you might as well just get used to your lot in life, because you have no control over who you are and what you can achieve. The victim cultivates feelings of helplessness and powerlessness, as it convinces you that there's nothing you can do to change your life's circumstances, because there's just something inherently defective about you. This personality is great at fostering depression.

Discovering that worry, perfectionism, depression and criticism all feed into anxiety disorders can be an eye-opener, but the more you study each of these sub-personalities, the more you will be able to dismantle them whenever they disguise themselves in your thinking.

Start by paying attention to occasions in which you feel anxious, panicky, depressed, self-critical, angry or otherwise upset. Then try to identify the negative or lie-based belief or thought underlying the emotion, as well as the sub-personality that is at work fostering this thought. What are you telling yourself whenever you feel down or anxious? Often there will be several lie-based thoughts contributing to the emotion(s), and while these can be difficult to separate and identify, it is a worthwhile endeavor that becomes easier with practice.

Write down these thoughts and challenge their truthfulness, keeping in mind the characteristics of each sub-personality so that you can recognize any tendencies to overestimate, catastrophize, overgeneralize and filter reality. To help determine whether a thought is true, ask yourself whether there is, or has been, evidence now or in the past to validate the truth of your current fearful/negative thought. Then, imagine if it were true, and ask yourself what would be the consequences if so. Often, you will find that your fears are more devastating than if what you feared were actually to come true!

For example, let's say that Lyme disease causes you heart palpitations, and every time you experience a palpitation, you fear that you are going to die of a heart attack. There is not, nor has there ever been, any evidence to validate the truthfulness of this thought, so you can discard it. Even if your cardiac dysfunction were serious, what is the worst that could happen to you? If you died, would it be so horrible? After all, you would cease to experience worry and pain, and perhaps you'd find yourself in a wonderful afterlife.

After you have identified the belief or lie behind the harmful thought and subjected it to the aforementioned Socratic questions, write down a positive counter-statement for it, so you have ammunition to combat the thought or belief every time it presents itself.

For instance, one of the common lies I used to tell myself is, "You'll never heal from Lyme disease. Why, just look at yourself. You've been treating this disease for a year and you aren't any better off than you were a year ago!" The counter-statement I wrote for this harmful belief was, "It can take several years to recover from this illness, and I should expect to get better, because I am young, strong and tenacious. Besides, God is ultimately in control of my healing, and if I think about it, I have had some improvements from a year ago. My thinking can easily become distorted with this illness, especially during periods when I experience herxheimer reactions."

While it may seem daunting to write down every deleterious thought and formulate a rebuttal for each one, you may be surprised to find that you tend to repeat the same thoughts, over and over, in your mind. So you won't have to come up with as many counter-statements as you might think. By taking a week to identify and combat the most pernicious of these lies, you can make significant progress in breaking down your entrenched sub-personalities. While this exercise may at first seem difficult to do, if you persevere, you will find it progressively easier to kick out the lies and thereby rid yourself of anxiety.

Connie Strasheim

Visualizations for Healing...Two Mind-Body Techniques that Cost only Fifteen Minutes a Day

Have you ever tried drawing pictures in your mind as you repeat healing affirmations? Requiring just a small investment of time, performing this technique can be a useful adjunct for treating Lyme disease.

While repeating positive affirmations alone can be beneficial for healing, research has shown that performing visualizations with the mind's eye as you speak affirmations is even more effective, as images combined with words are thought to be very powerful.

Following are a couple of techniques that have proven to be useful for healing a myriad of disorders. The first I learned from a psychotherapist trained to work with those with health challenges. The second one I developed, though it resembles other widely-used strategies. Once you have established a routine, these techniques take only fifteen to twenty minutes a day to perform.

Visualization Technique #1

Close your eyes. Make sure you are in a quiet room where you won't be disturbed. Sitting up in a chair is best, though you can do this while lying down, too. Clear your mind of distracting thoughts and pretend you are going on a journey inside of your body. Notice the organs, tissues, joints, muscles and bones and any other parts you can think of.

After you have spent a minute or two looking inside yourself, envision your brain. Consider all that it has done for you; what its role has been in keeping you alive and the complicated functions that it performs every day. Think about how difficult it must be for it to function under the stress of Lyme disease, but how it faithfully keeps on working for you.

This process may take a few minutes as you pause to reflect upon the brain's multiple functions. After you have done this, ask it what it needs from you, and pause again as you wait for an answer. You might discern words, or receive an impression. When I first did this, the first thought that came to my mind was, "I need you to stop being angry at me for malfunctioning."

Once you receive an answer from the brain, respond to whatever you hear. If they are angry or sad words, apologize to your brain for whatever you have lacked giving it, whether it is nutrients or compassion or gratitude. Then thank it for all that it has done for you and tell it that although it hasn't been able to perform as perfectly as you'd like, you understand that it has always done the best it can. In fact, its functioning has been marvelous, considering the multitude of toxins and emotional trauma that it has been exposed to. The human body fights for life, even when mistreated, and continues to persevere and function, even under the harshest of circumstances. Meditating upon this sobering thought can help you to appreciate your brain and other parts. Express gratitude, and especially towards your creator, for what your brain has done for you.

Now, move on to the next part of your body, whether it be your heart, foot or liver, repeating the above procedure. Do this for as many parts as you have time for and are able to visualize. The more, the better, but don't get overwhelmed. Whenever I perform this exercise, I instinctively gravitate towards spending more time in parts of my body where there is significant dysfunction, so listening to your intuition can be helpful.

This exercise can help you to recognize how wonderfully made you are, as it enables you to have compassion towards your body and to recognize its great potential to heal itself.

If you feel that your body has betrayed you in some way, or you are angry with yourself because you can't do the things that you used to, then this is an especially good exercise for you.

Connie Strasheim

Visualization Technique #2

Shut those peepers again, and once again envision your body, with all of its organs, tissues, muscles, bones, fluids and so on. This time, begin by speaking aloud an affirmation that follows the below pattern or some variation thereof.

"Immune system, you have been wonderfully made by God. I command you, in the name of Jesus Christ (I use the name of Jesus, in accordance with my spiritual beliefs and because I believe there is power in using His name), to produce white blood cells to go after borrelia burgdorferi and other pathogens in my body. I give you eyes to see this harmful bacteria, in all of its forms, whether spirochete, L-form or cyst, and eyes to see babesia, bartonella and (name other pathogens that you know you are infected with), and I command you to gobble these up, by the power of God's Holy Spirit." You might also command the pathogens to leave your body, affirming that they don't have any right to live in your cells.

After stating the affirmation, visualize your white blood cells engulfing pathogens or chasing them out of the body. Take the white blood cells to as many parts of the body as you can, including: your gastrointestinal tract, heart muscle, liver, brain, bone and anywhere else where it is easy for you to draw pictures with your mind's eye. To keep focused, repeat the above phrase aloud, continually and for each part of the body. Use as much detail as you can, though if it is difficult for you to envision certain parts of your body, that's okay, as long as you can produce an image, however vague, of white blood cells attacking pathogens.

Next, speak strength into each organ and system of the body. Begin with the brain, and speak healing to it, in accordance with what you intuit needs specific healing there. While you are speaking, envision it healthy and strong. For instance, I say to my brain, "God has declared you to be fearfully and wonderfully made. I therefore speak health into you now, and command you to produce the proper amount of chemicals and neurotransmitters for proper brain function. I command you to release all negative memories, pathogens and heavy metals and to stop taking my negative emotions and sending them to the body, where they produce illness. Be healed, by the power of God's holy name. Thank you, God."

Your mantra doesn't have to be this complicated. You might simply say, for instance, "To my adrenal glands, I command you to produce the proper amount of hormones for optimal health. Be healed."

The more convincingly you are able to recite your mantra, and the more detail you can add to the visualization, the greater may be the results you will reap from this exercise. If you aren't convinced by your affirmations at first, don't let this stop you, as your words spoken aloud may end up altering your thoughts over the long run.

You can combine the above exercises into one, so that you don't have to go through each part of your body twice, or you can alternate exercises when you don't have time to do both. Or you may prefer to always do one instead of the other.

While it isn't necessary and may be tedious to specify every single body part, you may want to use the following list to help you identify areas that need healing:

Brain
Skeleton
Muscles
Tendons, Ligaments, Joints
Central Nervous System
Lymphatic System
Heart, lungs and circulatory system
Kidneys
Digestive System (including stomach, small and large intestine, liver, gall bladder and pancreas)
Spleen
Adrenal glands and endocrine system (including the hypothalamus, pituitary gland, thymus, thyroid and sex organs)
Skin
Blood...and so on.

Connie Strasheim

Chapter 19

Strategies that Go Beyond the Conscious Mind

Releasing Emotional Trauma from the Body with Neuro-Emotional Technique

Did you know that the domain of healing emotional trauma resides not only in the brain but in the body, too? That's right; fixing emotional trauma isn't just a cognitive endeavor. It's physiological as well, and infections aren't the only things that break the body in Lyme disease. Stored emotional trauma does, too.

While a multitude of therapies exist to heal biochemical dysfunction caused by emotions, most focus upon cognitive approaches that give attention to the mind. However, according to a therapy called Neuro-Emotional Technique (www.netmindbody.com), emotional trauma, in the presence of a neurological deficit or problem with the body's

Connie Strasheim

energy flow, can cause physiopathological problems in the body. Or, in short, the trauma causes undesirable patterns of mind-body behavior, which NET terms "neuro-emotional complexes." These complexes are often triggered under stressful circumstances, creating an undesirable ritualistic response in the body and mind every time the stress is repeated.

Borrowing from a combination of multiple healing disciplines, including chiropractic, acupuncture, homeopathy, psychology and others, NET seeks to remove, via physical touch, the neuro-emotional complexes or, if you prefer, the dysfunctional mind-body patterns of behavior that are trapped in the body.

Touch therapy along key meridian points, spinal manipulation and inquiries into a patient's history of past trauma are all a part of this therapy, as is homeopathy, which is used to help awaken the body to the changes it needs to make. Psychological questioning helps inform the practitioner regarding the origins of potential neuro-emotional complexes in the body.

When it all comes together, the changes can be powerful, as reconditioning and release of unhealthy physiological processes takes place.

For example, let's say that every time you hear a door slam, your heart races because it reminds you of how, when you were a child, your uncle George used to slam doors before he entered your bedroom to smack you for fighting with your sister. NET effectively removes the trigger so that your heart ceases to pound every time you hear a door slam.

Neuro-Emotional Technique is useful for treating a myriad of disorders, including phobias, generalized anxiety, headaches, body aches, self-sabotaging behaviors and organ dysfunction. A couple of practitioners I interviewed stated that one or two sessions are usually sufficient to treat a particular issue, though occasionally a few more are warranted. Each session costs $150 or more. It isn't pocket change, but the therapy may be a worthwhile consideration for the Lyme disease sufferer for whom conscious or unconscious emotional trauma comprises an important part of his or her illness.

Reprogramming the Subconscious Mind to Rewire Your Cellular Behavior

Did you know that your belief system can keep you stuck in the slum of illness, no matter how many antibiotics you take?

Harmful or lie-based belief systems effectuate damaging changes in the ANS (autonomic nervous system) which governs the body's response to stress. When harmful thought patterns resulting from lie-based belief systems become pervasive, the ANS gets stuck in high-stress mode, which in turn suppresses the immune system, leading to illness.

While challenging dysfunctional beliefs on a conscious level can contribute towards keeping the ANS in a state of greater calm, the subconscious mind exerts a more powerful influence upon the body, and some of your deep-seated beliefs may remain known only to your subconscious mind. Hence, greater healing is often realized through therapies that bypass the conscious mind and go straight to the subconscious, where belief systems reside.

Suppose you tell yourself that you want to heal from Lyme disease and that you will in fact heal from Lyme disease, but you find yourself doubting despite your verbal affirmations. This is because your subconscious is quietly refuting your conscious decision. It might be telling you, "You won't heal because you don't deserve good things." Unlike the conscious mind, it doesn't articulate these words, but they are wrapped up within the cozy confines of dark belief, which becomes the driving force behind your body's ability to heal.

Don't despair. You can heal, even if your conscious desires conflict with your subconscious beliefs. Therapies that go beyond positive affirmations and counseling exist to help undo the destructive patterns that thrive below the conscious mind. These often don't make sense on a cognitive level but speak profoundly to the quiet, yet powerful subconscious.

Emotional Freedom Technique, The Healing Codes, Thought Field Therapy, Lightning Therapy, Neuro-Emotional Technique, Immune Response Therapy and Quantum Techniques are examples of therapies that help to rewire belief systems by going deeper than the conscious mind to tap into the power of the ANS and the subconscious. They offer hope to Lyme disease sufferers who feel that they have tried everything, from medication to counseling, to combat their depression and anxiety, and are a great resource for anyone who knows that their healing depends upon rewiring dysfunctional patterns of belief.

Chapter 20

The Moral of the Story

Lessons from the Food Stamp Office...Don't Buy into Lies about Who You Are

I enter the food stamp office, a sense of lowliness fitting me like the hole-in-the-knee jeans and black T-shirt I'm wearing. Along with my mussed-up hair, they suit me up well for this place, located in Denver's impoverished Five Points district. I figure I'll fit in better if I dress down. Forget the make-up and designer slacks.

I glance about the somber, crowded room. I have about two minutes to find a chair, before my postural-orthostatic tachycardia syndrome sets in, my heart starts racing and I'm forced to take deep breaths to keep my body oxygenated.

All of the chairs are occupied. I contemplate the linoleum floor. Not an ideal place to plop down, but a backache is more tolerable than breathing problems and chest pain.

I take a number from the reception as a tired-faced woman calls out, "Jorge, Jorge Rodriguez..."

Connie Strasheim

I peek at my number and then glance at the digital counter on the wall. Only fifty folks ahead of me.

I sit down and wince as pain shoots up my spine and into my right shoulder. Why must I do this every three months? Can't the government come up with a more efficient system? Having to show up by 8:00 A.M. for a potential 11:00 A.M. interview is nonsense!

I fold my legs beneath me, and ache swims through my body. I could crash right here on the linoleum floor. It's amazing how getting up early makes me feel as though I've got a hangover.

I want to scream at the food stamp people, "Don't you know that there are disabled people in here? Can't you provide enough chairs? Can't you just schedule everyone's interview so that we don't all have to be here at 8:00 A.M.? Do you have any idea how difficult it is for me to get up this early?"

I laboriously rise, heart racing as my blood pressure plummets, and approach the receptionist. "Excuse me...."

Behind the desk is a lady with heavy make-up who cuts me off, "Take a number and we'll be right with you."

"But I just want to turn in—"

"Sit down, and we'll call your number!"

"But you don't understand, I just want to turn in an application."

She glares at me. "We'll call your number."

I exhale, heart pounding. A large woman wearing a Security badge has made her way over to me, and she gives me the once-over as I move away from the reception desk. Just what I need. To get thrown out by Security for insisting on a civil conversation with the food stamp office authorities.

My spot on the floor has been stolen by a shaggy man, and I plop down beside the pay phone, the last section of linoleum offering a bit of wall for a backrest.

"Number one hundred twenty," one of the front desk sharks calls out.

I glance at my crumpled-up ticket. Why must I check it every time they call out a number? Can't I remember that I'm one hundred seventy-two? Boy, am I grouchy today. Then again, I'm always in a bad mood when I have to come here.

Rising early, the half-hour drive and then having to wait three hours for an interview are all annoying and a waste of time, but today I wonder if there's more to my irritation than these things.

In the set of plastic chairs across from me, a pale-faced woman snatches up her toddler, who shrieks as she plops him down beside her.

"Can't you be still for two minutes?" She scolds.

Next to her sits an older woman in a burka, and the folds of her garment envelop a napping baby. Her round, dark eyes seem to smile in sympathy at the pale woman, as the toddler jumps down from the chair again and stomps across the room.

Then, "Miguel, ven aquí!" (Miguel, come here!). The voice from the far end of the room belongs to a Hispanic woman, who seems to have the same problem as the white lady, with a boy who's obviously tired of waiting in the food stamp office.

The room is filled with lethargic faces, some wearing hints of animosity or irritation. A few people chat with their neighbors, and it's a colorful scene of men and women of all ages and more than just a few races and languages. A couple of women wear head coverings, the young men don baggy jeans and baseball caps, but nobody is dressed to the nines, and not a soul looks pleased to be here. Opposite me is a man with a graying beard, worn face and stained suit hanging about

Connie Strasheim

his insignificant frame. Why do so many of the older ones look shabby and unkempt? Are they homeless? What's the older man's story? What are any of these people's stories?

As I sit there, my shoulder throbbing, I realize that I am getting a glimpse, albeit it a very scarce one, into the life of the impoverished in the United States. And then it strikes me that it's not only the inconvenience of trekking to the food stamp office every three months which bothers me about coming here, but also the way I feel when I am here.

Even stranger, my choice of attire and lack of attention to my grooming fosters this attitude, even though consciously I know I don't need to feel this way.

It's such an ugly thing, shame. I know I am sick and cannot work, yet the sensation of inadequacy gnaws at me anyway, like a rat nibbling on my lifeline of self-esteem. That I have to request governmental assistance to pay for groceries, no matter the cause, keeps the tortuous feeling alive within me, even though most of the time it disguises itself as a vague uneasiness.

I am not lazy, and this is not my fault! I know this, so why, oh why, does it hurt me to come here? What could I have done differently in my life so that I wouldn't have ended up begging for food and housing as a young adult? Should I have saved more money? Should I have paid more attention to the dysfunction of my body? Would it have mattered?

Just being in this sad place, I am stripped of my dignity. I never thought I'd ask for charity in my life. And yet here I am, with all of society's forsaken and impoverished.

My eyes fall again upon the pallid lady with the toddler. Her countenance sags, and her eyes reflect despair. It isn't fair that we should all have to live like this. Was this the life any of us signed up for?

Yes, at least we have some kind of social services system in this country to care for those here with me. Praise God for that. But who in this room would have ever have said to himself as a child, "When I grow up, I want to be penniless and sponge off of the government for my daily bread?"

I concede that enduring this inconvenient process provides me with one hundred and fifty dollars every month to help pay for food. Since I eat organic and purchase supplements, my grocery bill comes closer to four hundred dollars a month, but the money helps, anyway.

Perhaps I need to say a prayer or chant some kind of mantra the next time I come to the food stamp office. A mantra that affirms my self-worth and counters the ridiculous notion that I ought to be ashamed for requesting governmental assistance. Although it's funny how, the minute I step out of the food stamp office and go into the bathroom to change into a blazer and slacks for my two P.M. Spanish class, like Superman in a phone booth, I end up leaving feeling like a totally different person. That is, worthy of my nice clothes and vocation as a teacher.

Amazing what a sense of purpose, as well as a change of scenery or clothes, will do to a person's inner dialogue. I wonder if it would be the same for my fellow food stamp companions. Or what about my partners in Lyme? Would a little financial assistance, purpose or a change of environment enable them to climb out of the tar pit of illness faster?

Don't judge yourself if you are poor, alone and disabled. You are not one of society's forsaken. You have just as much worth as the soul who has a million-dollar home and thriving career, no matter that you can't work and need governmental assistance. Don't be ashamed. It's not your fault you got sick. Don't fall into the trap that I used to fall into at the food stamp office and allow the circumstances of illness to deceive you into buying into a lie about yourself.

Connie Strasheim

For One Hour, I Didn't Have Lyme Disease...Forgetting Your Limitations and Forging Ahead

Have you ever known what it's like to forget you have Lyme disease? Have you ever had an experience that allowed you to believe that you were healthier than those around you, even though your symptoms suggested the contrary? For one hour, I did. That was when I decided to ascend a waterfall in the spectacular rainforest of Manuel Antonio, in Costa Rica. Oh, how liberating was that moment!

Brainwashed by nature's beauty and my sense of adventure, when I saw the magnificent waterfall, I quickly forgot about the weakness in my limbs, the heaviness in my chest, and any fear of my limitations. I knew I just had to see what the fall looked like from above.

"Is there a path to the top?" I asked the four tourists who were bathing in the pool below.

They looked at one other and then at the shiny, jagged rock on either side of the crystalline waterfall. "I don't think so," said one. "Anyway, it looks slippery."

Mesmerized by the moving water, I might as well not have asked the question. I dropped my backpack and in my flip-flops, began to ascend narrow, rocky ledges.

My legs trembled. I commanded them to be strong. Too much was at stake. Fear took a swipe at me as I briefly imagined falling.

I moved fast, my legs and body growing stronger as I grappled for hand and foot holds in the rock. Where there weren't any, tree branches lent me their limbs.

My breathing labored, I soon reached the top and raised my eyes to a stunning view of the rainforest and a series of cascades, each one spilling into its own little pool of water that flowed towards the waterfall I'd just climbed.

I plopped down into one of the pools, directly beneath the cascade, and pounding water provided a spectacular massage for my aching back. Then, as I stood above the other tourists, who were looking up at me with what seemed a mix of curiosity and amazement, a sense of triumph overcame me. I have Lyme disease and I did this!

I smiled inwardly. The climb wasn't difficult; neither was it long, but the physically stronger around me wouldn't attempt it, even when I beckoned them to join me at the top.

For one glorious moment, I wasn't sick. As a friend once said to me, "You don't have Lyme disease. You're just a person who has a few health challenges." Perhaps we could all use a waterfall experience every now and again to show us that we aren't handicapped, at least not in our minds.

Sauna Talk, Part One...Learning to Share Lyme Disease with the World

In Denver, Colorado, saunas are a friendly, colorful place. Strangers chat with one another and people do all sorts of bizarre things while sweating out toxins. I never knew that going to the sauna could be so interesting. This therapy has enabled me to have fascinating exchanges with folks of all colors, shapes, sizes and... relational bents.

My neck is often full of tension due to Lyme disease, and, at times, I need to give it a good crack. This usually happens at the most inopportune of moments, such as during church, amidst the silence of the pew. Since the sauna's a more discreet place than church to relieve my tension, (just as long as the sound of a popping spine isn't loud enough to draw the attention of others), I often take advantage of my time there to snap my vertebrae back into place.

Connie Strasheim

So one day, as I am heating up inside the sauna, I feel the need for some crack. I pull my chin towards my shoulder, stretching my neck, and as I do this, the vertebrae pop, loud enough for all the sauna go-er's to hear me. Whoops. I glance timidly about the wood-paneled room, but it seems nobody's flinched.

But then, beside me, "Wow, I wish I could do that!"

I turn to look at the middle-aged man, who looks a bit like the lobster I had for dinner last night. Draw attention to my disability, why don't you? I think, my face burning. Fortunately, red faces aren't outside the norm in a sauna.

"You have back trouble?" He asks.

No, I just have Lyme disease. And a slew of emotional trauma stored in my spine. "Yeah, just a bit."

"What's that from?"

I don't want to go into the Lyme spiel right now. I'm just not up for the rigamarole of questions that will inevitably follow. Stuff like, "Where do you think you got bit by a tick? What's the treatment for that?" And then (big cringe), "But you look so good!"

Nope, just can't deal with that today. Neither am I interested in four sweaty guys finding out fifteen fun facts about me and Lyme disease. It's good to inform others about this dastardly illness, but, sometimes, I just don't want to talk about it.

So I say, "Just life, I guess."

He nods, and I move my eyes to the hot coils in the corner. Conversation ended.

A few minutes later, I glimpse my new friend tapping his eyebrows. EFT! I know exactly what he's doing. Emotional Freedom Technique.

He's a brave one to do that in public. I wonder if he'll hit all the bio-meridian points: head, chin, chest, armpits....

I feel a twinge of guilt for my evil thought. The man obviously doesn't care what others think, unlike yours truly here, and I'm still embarrassed that he's pointed out my crack problem.

"Is that EFT you're doing?" I ask. What better way to cultivate intimacy in the sauna, than to delve into a person's innermost rituals! (Well, he started it.)

His face shifts a deeper shade of crimson. Or maybe it's just me. After all, the guy's been in this boiler room a good twenty minutes.

"Er, uh, yeah. So you know about EFT?"

I nod. Mission accomplished. He seems like a nice guy. Maybe I'll try to be kind now.

"Yeah, it's great stuff."

"I've never met anyone who knows EFT. How did you learn about it?"

Oh dear. Better watch where this thread goes. What do I say? "Well, actually, Lyme disease has made me into a basket case, and I learned about this technique during my passionate quest for mental health. Are you doing EFT for emotional stability, too?"

I say instead, "I like to read about alternative therapies."

He lifts a brow. "Oh, really? Why is that?"

Persistent, isn't he? "Just an interest of mine. So, what do you use EFT for?"

He suddenly looks bashful. "In the past, it healed me of a broken toe, and now it's ridding me of back pain and a bad knee."

Connie Strasheim

Fascinating. I hadn't known EFT to be useful for mending injuries. "How interesting. Well you look really good!" (I must be parroting something I've heard one too many times. So much that I'm now using the phrase inappropriately).

He faces me. I wish the sauna were bigger. "So you research health concepts, just for fun?"

Now I'm either going to have to tell a blatant lie or spill the Lyma beans. Sweat is doing a marathon down my cheeks. I wonder if it'll dry up white on my black shorts, from all the sea salt I've been taking lately. "Actually, I have a few health problems."

Compassionate eyes lock into mine. "Oh, I'm sorry. Have you found EFT to be helpful for you, too?"

"Yeah, it has. But it's okay. I'm learning a lot through treating my issues."

I'm getting a vibe like he's hankering to ask me what's wrong. I've got to squash the opportunity. It's nice he's interested, but I just can't deal with the questions today.

I've only been in the sauna twenty minutes, but it's time to go. Yeah, sometimes it's good to share this journey with others, but I'm not good about brevity and discretion and leaving unnecessary details out. If people really want to know, then I tell them, but today I don't feel like telling the whole sauna about this thing. And now, the only way I know how to control the conversation is to get out of the hot seat.

I grab my towel and stand, as dizziness assaults me. Leave it to my weak adrenal glands.

"You know, it's really getting warm in here. I've got to step out." I extend my hand. "It was so nice meeting you."

Surprise screws up his features as he shakes my hand. "Oh, yeah, likewise. My name's Mike, by the way."

"I'm Connie. See you later."

I open the door and the cool air of the gym evaporates the sweat on my face, and I think, maybe next time, when and if I see Mike, I'll tell him about Lyme disease. After all, people deserve to know about this illness. They need to know. In the meantime, I'll practice my discretionary skills so that I can tell him about it, without feeling as though I'm baring my soul to the whole sauna world, and pray for the patience to smile when he declares, "But you look so good!"

Sauna Talk Part II...Learning to Keep Life in Perspective

Didn't I tell you that the sauna is an interesting place for conversation? Okay, so I don't get out much, and I am probably too easily intrigued by my chat sessions in the hot room, but the verbal exchange I had today with a guy while sweating out toxins served to remind me of an important truth which I too easily forget.

So I'm in the sauna at 24-Hour Fitness, and a plump, dark-skinned African-American woman wearing a shower cap enters the sauna after me. She arranges herself across the wooden planks adjacent me. About ten minutes later, a tall, well-built man enters and sits down on the bench directly below her.

"That lady in the hot tub didn't believe me when I told her I be fifty-seven," he says.

I try not to stare at him. Fifty-seven? He doesn't look a day over forty, but isn't that the blessing of having dark skin? Not only that, but he's lean and muscular. No loose skin, no goose feet around the eyes, nothing to indicate that he's ever touched a greasy hamburger in his life. Heck, most people my age don't look that good.

Connie Strasheim

The shower cap lady chuckles. She sits up, removes her thick-rimmed glasses and rubs them clean with the edge of her towel. "Oh yeah? You tell her we be married for thirty years?"

You can't avoid eavesdropping on others' conversations in the sauna. You just have to be involved.

He sets his flip-flops next to his wife's. "Yeah, and then she tells me she be married for twenty. Couldn't believe that I be older than her."

He shifts his gaze towards me. In a friendly tone, says, "I think we've see you in here before."

No wonder he knows so much about the lady in the hot tub, which is just outside the sauna. He's a chatty one.

I say, "Yeah. I visit a couple of times a week. And you?"

The wife reclines against the planks again. Her husband says, "'Bout three times a week. Just the sauna. We got our own gym at home."

"Must be nice to have your own work-out space," I say, envy making an entrance into my emotional bank.

"Yeah, the kids like to use it when they come home. You got any of your own?"

"What, kids? No." I wipe my face with my towel, envisioning toxins soaking the rag. "How many do you have?"

"Three. We were gonna put a sauna and whirlpool in the house, too, but had to put the kids through college first."

Envy's presence is now official. The handsome, well-built man has a good marriage, three children and money to school them, with enough leftover change to build a gym in his house. He's got the whole package. And good health too, by the looks of him. Ah yes, it's the American dream, sitting smack in front of me.

I smile, thinking the expression a great veneer for my jealousy. "Well, I'd say you've done pretty well if you managed to get three kids through college." I almost add, "I can't even take care of myself." But then he'll ask why.

"That's beside the point. Those kids, they be a lot of work. You give up stuff for them."

Things like a whirlpool and sauna? Considering that I can't work because of Lyme disease, giving up a few luxury items to send three kids to college doesn't sound like such a huge sacrifice to me.

It's always like that, though. People I know complain about not having enough money for retirement or for a brand-new Volvo. There was a time when I worried about such stuff, too, but illness has knocked down my expectations. My needs now fall lower on Maslow's hierarchy. To even fathom being able to re-open a retirement account or one day purchase a new car is beyond me. Or a home of my own, since I had to give my condo back to the bank. No, I'm in survival mode. Just give me my daily bread and get me healed.

I nod. "I'm sure."

The man leans over to caress his wife's cheek. "How ya doin', Baby? Not heating up too much, are you?"

"I'm doing just fine, Honey."

Why can't I just rejoice in the good things that others have? Smile when it all works out for my neighbor? Admittedly, it's easier when I'm feeling happy and optimistic. On a day like today, though, when my body hurts, and I'm exhausted, there's no end to the negative thoughts. I might as well be envious of the crack in the sidewalk.

I glance at the man. What happy eyes he has! He deserves to do well. He obviously treats his wife with respect and probably does others, too. No wonder the kids made it through college. He raised them right.

Connie Strasheim

He shifts his weight on the bench. "Yeah, but you know, we lost the youngest last year."

What? He didn't really say that, did he? By now, a young man has joined us in the sauna. He sits adjacent me, so I can't see how the older man's comment has affected him.

Yes, indeed, he did say it. I don't squirm at the revelation, though, because there was an ease, a comfort about this guy that made it okay for him to tell me anything.

Suddenly, I felt I could do the same. Just tell him anything, no matter how profound, and it would result in an easy exchange of conversation between two strangers that weren't really strangers.

But I'm still not sure about his comment. It was spoken so nonchalantly. In an even tone, I say, "I'm sorry. What happened?"

The man doesn't look at me, but instead reclines next to his wife and places a rag over his forehead. In an equally even tone, says, "Took his own life. Last November."

Last November? As in, three months ago? Can I get a blue ribbon now for my judgmentalism? Yet, it isn't the first time that God has revealed to me that nothing is as it seems when it comes to others' lives. Just because theirs look so perfect from the outside. Just because I have Lyme disease, and it's taken my comfortable life from me, doesn't mean that I can compare my life to anyone else's. Not for a second.

Besides, what about the good things that Lyme disease has given me? No, I won't see these as long as I've employed Envy to show me what I lack, and isn't it good at its job on days when symptoms flare!

All the dumb thoughts vanish. "I'm really sorry. I can't fathom what it must be like to lose a child."

"Nothin' like it in the world."

I'm still not uncomfortable that he's shared this, but I wonder if the younger guy next to us is squirming.

"Do you believe your son is in a better place?" Never asked that question to a man I've only known for two minutes.

He doesn't answer, but sits up again. "Say, what's your name?"

"Connie."

"Connie, it's nice to meet you. My name's John, and this here is my wife, Rita."

Rita sits up. I rise to shake their hands. "Nice to meet you. Look, I'd love to talk with you more, but it's getting toasty in here."

I feel guilty for leaving the sauna, as though I'm trivializing this tender conversation, but my heart is walloping from the heat. I add, "May God bless you."

John says, "You believe in the Bible? That's good."

How did he know? "I do. I hope to see you again."

Warm eyes hold mine. "Likewise. You take care now."

"You, too."

And there's my lesson for the day. As envy tucks its tail between its legs and retreats from my mind, I think, Lyme disease isn't so bad. I think losing a child is probably a greater cross to bear. As I leave the gym, I wonder if I can go another minute without looking at the world through cracked lenses.

Connie Strasheim

Appendix: Spiritual Lessons Based on My Personal Belief in a God Who Heals

Born to Fly, but Stuck in Jail...Finding Freedom in a Life that Feels Confining

I used to be on an airplane eighteen days a month. Boy, how I still thirst for a nice jaunt around the planet! But never mind traveling and being on an airplane. We have all been born to fly, but oh how stubborn we are to spread our wings!

I recall the night when I first sensed I was ill. I still wore the fatigue of a fourteen-hour workday with United Airlines, even though I'd had three days to shake it off. Yet, I packed for my next grueling three-day trip, sure that another night's sleep would fix the heaviness and fog in my body. Little did I know that it was the last time I'd ever pack for a trip in my job as a flight attendant.

That night, I awakened, my heart walloping a hundred and fifty beats per minute. It wasn't a panic attack. I knew the difference. I dressed and went to the hospital emergency room, annoyed that I was now losing precious hours of rest before my long shift the following day. I couldn't call in sick, either. I'd already done that three times over the past year and had received a written warning regarding my absences. One more call-in and I'd be game for a suspension.

In the end, I didn't have to worry about it, because the sick call to my supervisor the following day soon became permission to take a long leave of absence.

In the first months following my mystery symptoms, a recurring dream assaulted me. In it, I am inside a jail cell, looking out at the world with all of its movement, color and energy and realizing that I can't participate in that world anymore. I watch people laugh and play and go about their day, while I remain trapped inside of my dark, dank, filthy cell. I pound on the walls as I scream and cry out to be

Connie Strasheim

freed, but my voice gets hoarse, and my arms grow weak as my cries fall on blackened walls. Helpless, I collapse onto the floor.

I often awakened to the grim feeling that my dream was for real. The morning sun would filter into my bright bedroom, but grief enfolded me in her black blanket. I was now in a prison called illness and couldn't participate in my former life anymore. I was serving a sentence of unknown duration without understanding what I'd done to deserve the incarceration. Not yet knowing what was wrong with me and how to get out of the cell put freedom on a vague, distant horizon. I didn't understand then that this pain was the beginning of what I would need to experience in order to grieve the life I'd lost and to find the courage to embrace a new one.

Three years later, I'm still prone to finding myself in jail. Not being able to work full-time, ski down a mountain, or have as much money as I'd like to spend leaves me feeling trapped, but it's not quite the same as before.

During my first months of Lyme disease hell, I often envisioned God, standing on the outside of my jail cell, dangling a key with the word "health" engraved upon it. If only I could come up with the magic word or deed he wanted from me, He'd unlock my cell and set me free into the world again.

After awhile, I stopped trying to figure it out, and improvements in my mental health enabled me to squash the false belief that my freedom was about an impossible jigsaw puzzle from my creator. Neither was it about attaining an absence of physical symptoms, but rather, a new state of mind.

Three years in the training camp of Lyme Disease Hell have now morphed my black iron prison into a soft little clay hut that has no lock and key, but rather, an open door. I can stay inside, where it's dark but safe, but I can also leave if I really want to. And on some days, I have been able to take tentative steps into the sunlight. On other days, I have even been able to spread my wings and soar into the treetops surrounding my hut.

Whenever I do, I realize that freedom resides not in my physical health, but in finding joy through all of life's circumstances. It is found in being able to smile even though I hurt. It lies in appreciating the beauty of who God has made me to be, instead of reproaching my body for not cooperating with me. It resides in responding calmly to traffic and the anger of others; in not worrying about being jobless and broke, but instead treasuring the time I have to care for myself. It lies in not lamenting what is no longer, but rejoicing in what is still there; in sharing a joke with friends instead of resenting their lack of understanding towards my illness, and in loving instead of waiting to be loved. It is in knowing that God loves me despite my imperfections, and that this journey of illness is not about Him locking me up inside of a prison and waiting for me to figure out the reason for my suffering. Rather, it's about setting me free so that, whatever my circumstances, wherever I am, I can soar like an eagle and fly, even if I am never 100% healed in my physical body again. You can fly, too, if you have the will, but you must first know that your prison has an open door.

The Redemptive Potential of Illness and the Power of God to Make it Happen

If only life could be perfect. If only health, wealth, love and every whimsy of ours ended up in our favor. If only happiness were constant, joy abundant, and excitement plentiful. If only there were no more tears, no more rage, sadness, or depression. No more poverty, no more broken hearts, bodies and minds. Who hasn't wondered why Earth cannot be Eden? Why God won't right all the wrongs? The God of Christianity, whom I follow, sure isn't interested in making life on earth perfect for His followers. Whether or not you believe in my god, you may yet agree that our creator, or the universe, isn't into comfort or into giving us all things that we call good. No, God isn't into helping us achieve the American dream, though He may bestow some of its benefits upon us.

In fact, when it comes to His little creatures that he so professes to love, He really lets the crap hit the fan. He allows death and devastation and tears aplenty. He permits us to be rent and reviled, broken and struck down, battered, bruised and beaten to the ground. And just when we think we can't handle another devastation, we are broadsided by tragedy once again. And in the name of love, He allows it all. Concentration camps in Nazi Germany, genocide in Sudan and AIDS all over the place. Then of course, Lyme disease, and year upon year of fatigue, depression and a life void of ambitious activity, recreation and functional relationships.

This isn't to say that all of this devastation was in His original plan. Christians would say that it wasn't, but that tragedy is the price paid for free will and must exist in order for God's creatures to be able to have the freedom to love. But is it worth the price of a planet rife with murder, starvation, sickness and every conceivable horror we can imagine?

My god apparently thinks so.

Yes, and He fixes some of it here on earth, but not all of it, and though rationally we may understand why not, the eternal question of suffering leaves no answers that really satisfy the aching gut of a Lyme disease sufferer. So I won't pretend to have solutions, but instead will share tidbits of light that God has given me through my journey with Lyme disease.

I haven't fully wrapped my mind around the following, and don't think that because I can say it, I can live it or even believe it much of the time. Yet something about it demands acknowledgement, though remember, I'm mostly just a messenger with words.

No, God isn't about making it all pleasant and perfect. What He is about is redemption—that is, taking the bad and bringing good from it, because redemption is one of the most spectacular manifestations of love's power. And God is big on love. For Him, love allows another to suffer, and often such suffering must be present in order for love to display its beautiful and majestic plumage. It is a kingdom and a power more formidable than anything on earth, and that power lives in God, and is God.

And redemption is His method. Consider the following:

It is wonderful to receive a soft, velvety red rose, but awe-inspiring to contemplate the paradox of a rose bush and to know that the plethora of soft, beautiful flowers grew from stiff branches with sharp thorns.

It is heart-warming to see a man who has compassion towards the poor, but soul-moving to discover that he was once a starving orphan in Africa and now feeds millions by the grace that was once given to him.

For those of us who are Christians, it is horrible to think that God's Creation murdered Jesus Christ, the One who gave It life, and yet paradoxical that the most atrocious act committed in the history of mankind was used to bring eternal life to that Creation.

It is tragic to watch a Lyme disease sufferer lose his or her home, career and health. Illness, poverty and the rest are devastations that many people around us don't have to suffer. That we must endure these things while others don't feels like punishment, a curse and all that is wrong with the world, but God would see it as ripe ground for redemption; as an opportunity for love to reach its powerful arms around our pain and transform it. Even if you don't believe in God, you can still believe in the redemptive power of illness. Growth is the fruit of suffering if you allow it to be, and illness has a blessed way of stuffing all of your life's demons in your face so that you have no choice but to face them or forget about ever walking in health again.

It forces you to find good in a life that feels too tragic to be true and to rely upon a higher truth to help you see that what really matters is getting rid of the internal darkness, so that light can shine through. If you have dreams, if you have hopes, and if you believe you deserve to be healthy and loved and have the capacity to do great things for the world, then you will face your demons, because you know you won't ever heal if you don't. Furthermore, in the absence of activity and recreation, the ghosts become a little harder to ignore.

Connie Strasheim

In my humble opinion, this is what God is about. Finding the greatest garbage heaps, delving into the darkest tar pits, searching far and wide for the world's greatest sob stories, so that He can demonstrate love's unfathomable power to transform. And the muckier the tar pit, the greater the opportunity for His light to shine.

Of course, it's not an overnight thing. For those of us who believe in God and His ability to redeem us, the light of His power upon us often feels no brighter than a candle, and the changes within, like snail steps towards some unreachable horizon. We expect our hearts to change by two degrees, if at all. Indeed, redemption from our inner darkness often feels like a pipe dream reserved for a few lucky saints and the afterlife.

Yet, I believe that it is far from what God hopes to do with us. He is saddened, I think, that we have resigned ourselves to a life of baby steps towards a tolerable existence.

If you are anything like me, after reading this, you might stage a beat-up session with yourself, wondering why, if the aforementioned is true, you aren't drinking more deeply of the juice of redemption. Or you may turn your fists toward God and ask Him, Why, after so many years of suffering, do you still feel the same?

Once, when I got into the boxing ring with God, He reminded me that healing isn't just about what I am supposed to do with my demons, but what I am supposed to believe that He will do with them, because it is He who empowers me to change. He reminded me that I need to stop trying to actualize myself by my own power, to cease believing that I can raise myself from the dead, and to quit drawing up ridiculous schedules and time sheets by which I measure my progress.

Don't think that this means that I know how to "let go and let God." That pious little phrase rubs me the wrong way because, ninety percent of the time, I don't get what it means. Fortunately, God is lowering that percentage, little by little, as I patiently and impatiently wait through circumstances that are too tiresome and dull for my liking, although I still take comfort in the Bible verse, "For it is God who works in you to will and to do..."

Through it, I hear God saying, "I'll make it so that you will want to think and do what is best for your heart and Mine. I'm going to help you to change your thinking so that you may receive My prosperity, not the world's." And then, with the enthusiasm of an exuberant child, "Oh please, just let me! Let me!"

I seldom see God as a child, but in a flash of revelation I feel His excitement, just like that of a child before a pile of hidden treasures. He can't wait to dig through it, in order to uncover the jewel of His love, which has been buried by years of the world's garbage but which, if allowed, can yet be unearthed and polished to sparkle like never before.

Sparkle so that I can have compassion upon others who are ill, broken and battered, as I come to realize that I am greatly loved by my god. The ironic thing is that He is using, and will continue to use, my tragedies as tools to remove the filth and stinky refuse from the jewel. Love is that important, and when it comes to Creation receiving the Universe's highest joy, my god will allow anything to accomplish His purposes. Anything at all.

Finding Peace and Joy through Pain and Suffering

I used to think that peace was something God automatically bestowed upon anyone who spent time in prayer. Or that it was a nice by-product of having a happy upbringing and enough serotonin in the brain. My journey with illness, however, has taught me that peace and its oft-companion joy are, paradoxically, found through pain and suffering.

Perhaps it's because Lyme disease is teaching me to appreciate things that I am able to do now but which I could not do earlier on in my healing journey. Things like taking hour-long walks without heaving from exhaustion or laughing without falling short of breath. Or deciding to be grateful for what is instead of what isn't, and finding the

Connie Strasheim

good in a situation rife with difficulty because if I don't, I'll never be well again. It's quite an ultimatum, but I've found that more is at stake when you are ill and a pessimist than when you are relatively healthy and choose to see the glass as half-empty.

Or maybe it's because illness has a remarkable way of showing me that true peace cannot be built upon the shifting sands of circumstance. Take worldly prosperity away and upon what foundation do you build your joy? Illness is forcing me to find other sources, particularly in the spiritual realm.

Finally, my compassion is growing towards others who ail and ache. Requisite for relating to another's brokenness, suffering is allowing me to love others more deeply and to help them through their trials, thereby rewarding me with a few more P & J sandwiches.

This doesn't mean I like that life is engineered this way, because I'm not the Dalai Lama or Jesus Christ, and it's hard to live out what I know. A big part of me wonders why peace and joy can't just be bestowed upon me like fairy dust, and why everything good and lasting must have a price tag attached to it.

Yet, when I am able to think like a mature adult, I realize that peace is not found in a life of comfort and in the fulfillment of all my whims. Sometimes, it is found in the counter-intuitive place of pain, and in loss instead of gain.

Learning to Long for God, First and Foremost

"Your health isn't what you really want, above all things."

What? If someone had said these words to me off-handedly, as I was driving to the gas station or shopping for squash, I might have regarded them as nonsense. Who would ever say such a thing? Of course I want my health! I desire to be well more than anything else in the world.

And I've asked God a million times to heal me, because I believe He can do it in an instant, whether supernaturally or using man's medicine. At times, I've even pleaded and begged and soaked my sofa with tears, using up all of the toilet rolls in the house, as the faucet of my eyes ran on endlessly.

I used to wonder why He wasn't moved by my large emotions. What did I need to do in order for Him to change His mind about my plight? Did I need to believe Him more for my healing? How much longer before I'd learn whatever I was supposed to learn and He'd give me my health back?

All this devising, imploring, bargaining and hand-wringing with God, and you would think that the world was going to end if I weren't well by tomorrow. But seriously, in moments of irrationality, I couldn't imagine another year of this biochemical hell, let alone a lifetime. How could pain and fatigue ever be God's long-term plan for anyone? I can understand a year or two of illness, so that He might teach me a thing or two about how to take care of myself and have compassion towards others. But to be housebound and helpless, without any kind of work, ambition or activity to sustain me, for years and years, and to exist like a motionless mushroom in the ground...No, my sovereign god wouldn't allow that, would He?

All speculation aside, I guess I don't believe that this nightmare scenario is His will for those who suffer from chronic illness, but I stupidly yet ask why, if this is true, He won't heal me or others that I know. As if the riddle is ever going to be solved in this lifetime!

Lying in bed one morning at 11:00 AM, with my limbs aching, joints cracking and brain fried like my morning eggs, I went through my question checklist again with God, just as I have done a thousand times before, but changing the words around a little for conversation's sake.

I said, "So why must I feel like crap, Lord? Is this all you have for me? I'm thirty-one and I awaken every morning feeling like I'm eighty-one." (No, I don't know what eighty-two feels like, but my dad is sixty-

Connie Strasheim

one and is more active than I am. So I figure that tacking on a couple of decades puts me at a truer biological age, if I distort reasoning a bit and judge according to how I feel).

In my inability to move from beneath the covers, and after about fifteen minutes of questions that were more like accusations, I realized the futility of the rigamarole. Did I really expect a valid answer to the never-before completely answered question of suffering? Did I honestly expect to be the first human being to whom God would give such a revelation?

So I resigned myself to shutting off my own thoughts to listen to Him. I mean, really listen. Today I was going to give Him all the time He needed, instead of the normal ten or thirty minutes I offer Him every day during my morning quiet time. I'm sure that I shut out His wisdom when I put Him on my schedule.

I closed my eyes, and after a few minutes, knowledge that has been stored somewhere in the deep, dusty archives of my mind began to surface and take shape. Knowledge that most of the time stays buried in my gray matter or which surfaces briefly but frequently as a superficial statement of truth that never quite makes it to the heart. I've heard it a hundred times before, but most of the time, I don't comprehend it. Its edges touch my soul only when I am quiet and still and desperate for truth.

So here it was again. I didn't want to believe it at first. Most of the time, I don't. Not in my heart, anyway.

So what? You ask.

Well...it's just...the grass isn't necessarily greener on the other side of illness. No, it's God who makes my lawn green, regardless of my circumstances, and if I had to choose between physical health and God, it's God that I really need and want.

Funny how my quiet time with God had transformed this knowledge once again from trite speculation into spirit-filled wisdom, spreading it as a revelation throughout my cells, only because I had chosen to sit and be quiet before Him, long enough for Him to speak, on His terms.

Too often, my daily prayers, when scheduled and blithe, resemble thirty minutes with a therapist who happens to be called the creator of the universe. This creator exists to bless my will and fulfill my dreams and, as such, cannot be my friend, father or true companion. He can only be my genie or my Santa Claus. With this perspective, how could I ever think that His presence alone would be sufficient for my joy? After all, who cares about Santa if he doesn't have a gift to drop down the chimney? Today, God seemed to be reminding me that true life is found whenever I give Him the time of day to be something besides my toy dispenser and whenever I cease to believe that my freedom is found in the functioning of my limbs.

As I vaguely touched this reality with my fingertips, I held it in my mind for as long as I could—perhaps five minutes or so. By the time I rose from my knees, however, it had already begun its retreat into my visceral gut, where it would prod me in moments thereafter, to remind me that my lot in life doesn't matter a fraction as much as does my connection to God.

I don't pretend a level of sanctification that is currently beyond me. I still need the circumstantial crutches of this earth to contribute to my well-being, yet I have to wonder if being housebound for years could actually bring me greater joy than being street-bound with ambitions aplenty and the resources to fulfill them. Yeah, perhaps if I were Jesus Christ or the Apostle Paul.

Then again, if forty-five minutes listening to my lord could convince me that He is really what I want, far and above my physical health, then what would this much time, spent in humility with Him every day, do for my belief system? Would I still crave health as I do now? Is it possible that I could find greater peace in that quiet, housebound place of desperation than in the frenetic life of stimulus that physical health demands?

Connie Strasheim

Why Won't God Heal Me?

In the Bible, Jesus says that the prayer of faith will heal the sick, but I have to wonder what he meant. Especially when I know Lyme disease sufferers who profess to follow the god of Christianity, claim the Scripture's promises, and yet spend year after year bedridden or housebound due to illness. They pray, they believe God for healing, but they remain ill. You might be one of these. I am, too, and while I know that God is healing me, I'm not there yet.

So I often present the challenge to God. If what Jesus says is true, then why must I, why must anyone, spend years in relentless pain and fatigue? To the Pat-Answer folk, I say, spare me your answers. I already know what the Bible says about suffering, but God's truths are sometimes elusive to the heart when the body screams out in pain, no matter that the mind and the spirit know better.

These smug souls might be happy to know that the Bible comforts me anyway, even though I don't believe that I can take my god's word literally, and that trying to grasp onto any explanation of why not is like wearing a bad pair of shoes that don't fit properly. And although my toes writhe inside of those shoes, I wear them anyway because I need something to stand in, and if I move around in them long enough, maybe I can adjust to them.

Adjust to the promises that have exceptions, to the explanations and seeming contradictions. Yes, Jesus heals, but not always! Or pick your favorite shoe, so that you'll have something to walk around in. I hadn't found a pair I felt good in, until recently. A pair that would move me to great distances, or a pair that would leave me comfortable. But before I found my current set of sneakers, I tried on some of the following shoes of explanation:

a) God heals but it doesn't mean right away. Heck, it might mean in the afterlife.

b) He didn't mean that the prayer of faith would always heal. No, God isn't into formulas.

c) Since Scripture says that faith is required to heal the sick, maybe I don't have enough faith. Then again, how much faith is enough? I've witnessed miraculous healing. I know God is able and willing to do it, and can accomplish it in an instant.

d) Jesus healed during biblical times to demonstrate God's love to humanity. There's no point in Him doing it now, since He's already proven His love through Christ's death on the Cross.

e) The Bible just can't be taken literally.

f) The healing Jesus speaks of isn't physical.

g) God wants me to love Him for who He is, and not His gifts.

h) God wants to teach me a lesson, such as that He's not a vending machine.

i) Put your favorite theological point here.

Fortunately, as of late, I've put on another pair of shoes. These fit better than the other ones because I feel that they have been tailor-made to my situation and are not the product of any frustrated musings (though I still get blisters from them sometimes).

Whenever I wear them well, I know that it is God's will for me, for any of His children, to be healed, but that it can't always be done in an instant. I know that God could heal my physical body with just a swift breath of divine air, but it wouldn't matter as long as much work remains to be done in my spirit. And that inner work is something I'm supposed to be actively involved in, because it's a job involving my mind and will, and asking for the intercession of a holy hand would also mean asking for my free will to be snatched out from under me.

Connie Strasheim

Indeed, God could heal my physical body right now, but I might relapse, as long as other parts of me need work.

If you are like me, you may go through stages when no pair of shoes fits right. Even when you find ones that work for you, you may find yourself taking them off anyway, because the cool grass feels better beneath your feet than a couple of hard soles. Indeed, you might decide that it's preferable to run around barefoot, instead of asking why God won't heal you now, because you know that someday, in the not-so-distant future, your Eden of perfect health will be granted to you. In the meantime, you can savor the small gains that bring you every day closer to its garden.

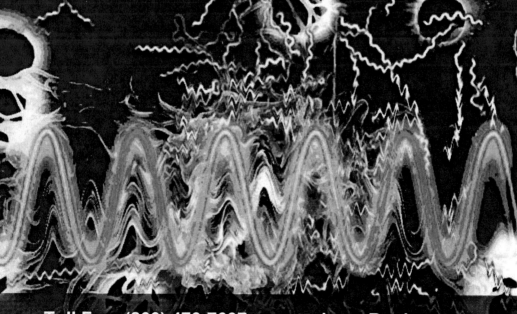

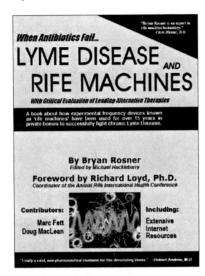

Book • $35

When Antibiotics Fail: Lyme Disease And Rife Machines, With Critical Evaluation Of Leading Alternative Therapies

By Bryan Rosner
Foreword by Richard Loyd, Ph.D.

There are enough books and websites about what Lyme Disease is and which ticks carry it. But there is very little useful information for people who actually have a case of Lyme Disease that is not responding to conventional antibiotic treatment. Lyme Disease sufferers need to know how to get better, not how to identify a tick.

This book describes how electromagnetic frequency devices known as rife machines have been used for over 15 years in private homes to successfully fight Lyme Disease. Also included are evaluations of more than 20 conventional and alternative Lyme Disease therapies, including:

- Homeopathy
- IV and oral antibiotics
- Mercury detox.
- Hyperthermia / saunas
- Ozone and oxygen
- Samento®
- Colloidal Silver
- Bacterial die-off detox.

- Colostrum
- Magnesium supplementation
- Hyperbaric oxygen chamber (HBOC)
- ICHT Italian treatment
- Non-pharmaceutical antibiotics
- Exercise, diet and candida protocols
- Cyst-targeting antibiotics
- The Marshall Protocol®

Many Lyme Disease sufferers have heard of rife machines, some have used them. But until now there has not been a concise and reliable source to explain how and why they work, and how and why other therapies fail. In the book you will learn that rife machine therapy offers numerous advantages over antibiotic therapy, including sustained effectiveness, affordability, convenience, autonomy from the medical establishment, and avoidance of candida complications.

The Foreword for the book is by Richard Loyd, Ph.D., coordinator of the annual Rife International Health Conference. The book takes a practical, down-to-earth approach which allows you to learn about:

> "This book provides life-saving insights for Lyme Disease patients."
>
> **- Richard Loyd, Ph.D.**

- Why rife machines work after other therapies fail, with analysis of antibiotics.
- Rife machine treatment schedules and sessions.
- The most effective rife machines: High Power Magnetic Pulser, EMEM Machine, Coil Machine, and AC Contact Machine.
- Explanation of the "herx reaction" and why it indicates progress.
- Evaluation of leading alternative therapies.
- Antibiotic categories and classifications, and which antibiotics are most efficacious.
- What it feels like to use rife machines – discover the steps to healing!

Paperback book, 8.5 x 11", 203 pages, $35

The Top 10 Lyme Disease Treatments: Defeat Lyme Disease With The Best Of Conventional And Alternative Medicine

By Bryan Rosner
Foreword by James Schaller, M.D.

This information-packed book identifies ten cutting-edge conventional and alternative Lyme Disease treatments and gives practical guidance on integrating them into a comprehensive treatment plan that maximizes therapeutic benefit while minimizing side effects.

This book was not written to replace Bryan Rosner's first book (*Lyme Disease and Rife Machines*). Instead, it was written to complement that book, offering Lyme sufferers many new foundational and supportive treatments to use during the recovery process. New treatments and information in this book include:

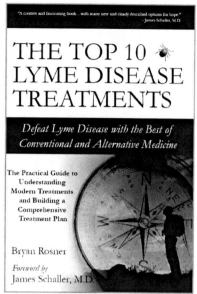

"A creative and fascinating book...with many new and clearly described options for hope."
- James Schaller, M.D.

THE TOP 10
LYME DISEASE
TREATMENTS

Defeat Lyme Disease with the Best of Conventional and Alternative Medicine

The Practical Guide to Understanding Modern Treatments and Building a Comprehensive Treatment Plan

Bryan Rosner

Foreword by
James Schaller, M.D.

Book • $35

- Systemic enzyme therapy, which helps detoxify tissues and blood, reduce inflammation, stimulate the immune system, and kill Lyme Disease bacteria.
- Lithium orotate, a powerful yet all-natural mineral (belonging to the same mineral group as sodium and potassium) capable of profound neuroprotective activity.
- Thorough and extensive coverage of a complete Lyme Disease detoxification program, including discussion of both liver and skin detoxification pathways. Specific detoxification therapies such as liver cleanses, bowel cleanses, the Shoemaker Neurotoxin Elimination Protocol, sauna therapy, mineral baths, mineral supplementation, milk thistle, and many others. How to reduce and control herx reactions.
- Tips and clinical research from James Schaller, M.D.
- A detailed look at how to properly utilize antibiotics during a rife machine treatment campaign.

"Bryan Rosner thinks big and this new book offers big solutions."
- James Schaller, M.D.

"Another ground-breaking Lyme Disease book."
- Jeff Mittelman, moderator of the Lyme-and-rife group

"Brilliant and thorough."
- Nenah Sylver, Ph.D.

- Wide coverage of the Marshall Protocol, including an in-depth description of its mechanism of action in relation to Lyme Disease pathology. Also, the author's personal experience with the Marshall Protocol over 3 years.
- An explanation of and new information about the Salt / Vitamin C protocol.
- Hot-off-the-press information on mangosteen fruit (not to be confused with mango) and its many benefits, including antibacterial, anti-inflammatory, and anti-cancer properties.
- New guidelines for combining all the therapies discussed in both of Rosner's books into a complete treatment plan. Brief and articulate with step-by-step instructions for healing.
- Also includes updates on rife therapy, cutting-edge supplements, political challenges, an exclusive interview with Willy Burgdorfer, Ph.D. (discoverer of Lyme), and much more!

Do not miss this top Lyme Disease resource. Discover new healing tools today!

Paperback book, 7 x 10", 367 pages, $35

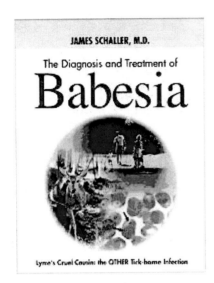

JAMES SCHALLER, M.D.

The Diagnosis and Treatment of

Babesia

Lyme's Cruel Cousin: the OTHER Tick-borne Infection

Book • $35

The Diagnosis and Treatment of Babesia: Lyme's Cruel Cousin – The Other Tick-Borne Infection

By James Schaller, M.D.

Do you or a loved one experience excess fatigue? Have you ever had unusually high fevers, chills, or sweats? You may have Babesia, a very common tick-borne infection. Babesia is often found with Lyme Disease and, like all tick-borne infections, is rarely diagnosed and reported accurately.

The deer tick which carries Lyme Disease and Babesia may be as small as a poppy seed and injects a painkiller, an antihistamine, and an anticoagulant to avoid detection. As a result, many people have Babesia and do not know it. Numerous forms of Babesia are carried by ticks - this book introduces patients and health care workers to the various species that infect humans and are not routinely tested for by sincere physicians.

Dr. Schaller, who practices medicine in Florida, first became interested in Babesia after one of his own children was infected with it. None of the elite pediatricians or child specialists could help. No one tested for Babesia or considered it a possible diagnosis. His child suffered from just two of these typical Babesia symptoms:

- Significant Fatigue
- Coughing
- Dizziness
- Trouble Thinking
- Fevers
- Memory Loss

- Chills
- Air Hunger
- Headache
- Sweats
- Unresponsiveness to Lyme Treatment

With 374 pages, this book is the most current and comprehensive book on Babesia in the English language. It reviews thousands of articles and presents the results of interviews with world experts on the subject. It offers you top information and broad treatment options, presented in a clear and simple manner. All treatments are explained thoroughly, including their possible side effects, drug interactions, various dosing strategies, pros/cons, and physician experiences.

"Once again Dr. Schaller has provided us with a much-needed and practical resource. This book gave me exactly what I was looking for."

- Thomas W., Patient

Finally, the book also addresses many other aspects of practical medical care often overlooked in this infection, such as treatment options for managing fatigue. Plainly stated, this book is a must-have for patients and health care providers who deal with Lyme Disease and its co-infections. Dr. Schaller's many years in clinical practice give the book a practical angle that many other similar books lack. Don't miss this user-friendly resource!

Paperback book, 7 x 10", 374 pages, $35

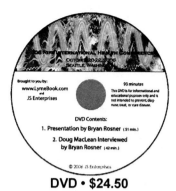

DVD • $24.50

Annual Rife International Health Conference DVD (93 Minutes)

Bryan Rosner's Presentation and Interview with Doug MacLean

The Official Rife Technology Seminar Seattle, WA, USA

If you were unable to attend the Rife International Health Conference, this DVD is your opportunity to watch two of the presentations that took place at the conference:

Presentation #1: Bryan Rosner's Sunday morning talk entitled *Lyme Disease: New Paradigms in Diagnosis and Treatment - the Myths, the Reality, and the Road Back to Health.* (51 minutes)

Presentation #2: Bryan Rosner's interview with Doug MacLean, in which Doug talked about his experiences with Lyme Disease, including the incredible journey he undertook to invent the first modern rife machine used to fight Lyme Disease. Although Doug's journey as a Lyme Disease pioneer took place 20 years ago, this was the first time Doug has ever accepted an invitation to appear in public. This is the only video available where you can see Doug talk about what it was like to be the first person ever to use rife technology as a treatment for Lyme Disease. Now you can see how it all began. Own this DVD and own a piece of history! (42 minutes)

Lymebook.com has secured a special licensing agreement with JS Enterprises, the Canadian producer of the Rife Conference videos, to bring this product to you at the special low price of $24.50. Total DVD viewing time: 1 hour, 33 minutes. We have DVDs in stock, shipped to you within 3 business days.

Price Comparison (should you get the DVD?)

Cost of attending the recent Rife Conference (2 people):
Hotel Room, 3 Nights = $400
Registration = $340
Food = $150
Airfare = $600
Total = $1,490

Cost of the DVD, which you can view as many times as you want, and show to family and friends:
DVD = $24.50

Bryan Rosner Presenting on Sunday Morning In Seattle

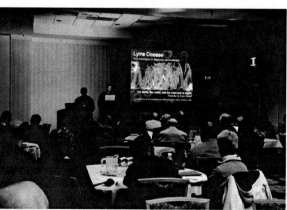

**DVD
93 Minutes
$24.50**

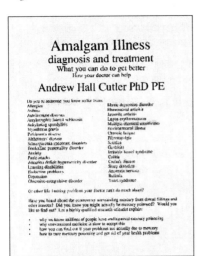

Book • $35

Amalgam Illness, Diagnosis and Treatment: What You Can Do to Get Better, How Your Doctor Can Help

By Andrew Cutler, PhD

This book was written by a chemical engineer who himself got mercury poisoning from his amalgam dental fillings. He found that there was no suitable educational material for either the patient or the physician. Knowing how much people can suffer from this condition, he wrote this book to help them get well. With a PhD in chemistry from Princeton University and extensive study in biochemistry and medicine, Andrew Cutler uses layman's terms to explain how people become mercury poisoned and what to do about it. Mercury poisoning can easily be cured with over-the-counter oral chelators – this book explains how.

In the book you will find practical guidance on how to tell if you really have chronic mercury poisoning or some other problem. Proper diagnostic procedures are provided so that sick people can decide what is wrong rather than trying random treatments. If mercury poisoning is your problem, the book tells you how to get the mercury out of your body, and how to feel good while you do that. The treatment section gives step-by-step directions to figure out exactly what mercury is doing to you and how to fix it.

"Dr. Cutler uses his background in chemistry to explain the safest approach to treat mercury poisoning. I am a physician and am personally using his protocol on myself."

- Melissa Myers, M.D.

Sections also explain how the scientific literature shows many people must be getting poisoned by their amalgam fillings, why such a regulatory blunder occurred, and how the debate between "mainstream" and "alternative" medicine makes it more difficult for you to get the medical help you need.

This down-to-earth book lets patients take care of themselves. It also lets doctors who are not familiar with chronic mercury intoxication treat it. The book is a practical guide to getting well. Sample sections from the book:

- Why worry about mercury poisoning?
- What mercury does to you – symptoms, laboratory test irregularities, diagnostic checklist.
- How to treat mercury poisoning easily with oral chelators.
- Dealing with other metals including copper, arsenic, lead, cadmium.
- Dietary and supplement guidelines.
- Balancing hormones during the recovery process.
- How to feel good while you are chelating the metals out.
- How heavy metals cause infections to thrive in the body.
- Politics and mercury.

This is the world's most authoritative, accurate book on mercury poisoning.

Paperback book, 8.5 x 11", 226 pages, $35

Hair Test Interpretation: Finding Hidden Toxicities

By Andrew Cutler, PhD

Hair tests are worth doing because a surprising number of people diagnosed with incurable chronic health conditions actually turn out to have a heavy metal problem; quite often, mercury poisoning. Heavy metal problems are easy to correct. Hair testing allows the underlying problem to be identified – and the chronic health condition often disappears with proper detoxification.

Hair Test Interpretation: Finding Hidden Toxicities is a practical book that explains how to interpret Doctor's Data, Inc. and Great Plains Laboratory hair tests. A step-by-step discussion is provided, with figures to illustrate the process and make it easy. The book gives examples using actual hair test results from real people.

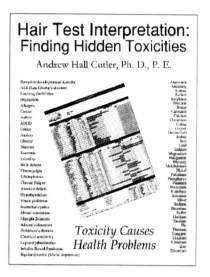

Hair Test Interpretation: Finding Hidden Toxicities

Andrew Hall Cutler, Ph. D., P. E.

Toxicity Causes Health Problems

Book • $35

One of the problems with hair testing is that both conventional and alternative health care providers do not know how to interpret these tests. Interpretation is not as simple as looking at the results and assuming that any mineral out of the reference range is a problem mineral.

Interpretation is complicated because heavy metal toxicity, especially mercury poisoning, interferes with mineral transport throughout the body. Ironically, if someone is mercury poisoned, hair test mercury is often low and other minerals may be elevated or take on unusual values. For example, mercury often causes retention of arsenic, antimony, tin, titanium, zirconium, and aluminum. An inexperienced health care provider may wrongfully assume that one of these other minerals is the culprit, when in reality mercury is the true toxicity.

"This new book of Andrew's is the definitive guide in the confusing world of heavy metal poisoning diagnosis and treatment. I'm a practicing physician, 20 years now, specializing in detoxification programs for treatment of resistant conditions. It was fairly difficult to diagnose these heavy metal conditions before I met Andrew Cutler and developed a close relationship with him while reading his books. In this book I found his usual painful attention to detail gave a solid framework for understanding the complexity of mercury toxicity as well as the less common exposures. You really couldn't ask for a better reference book on a subject most researchers and physicians are still fumbling in the dark about."
- **Dr. Rick Marschall**

So, as you can see, getting a hair test is only the first step. The second step is figuring out what the hair test means. Andrew Cutler, PhD, is a registered professional chemical engineer with years of experience in biochemical and healthcare research. This clear and concise book makes hair test interpretation easy, so that you know which toxicities are causing your health problems.

Paperback book, 8.5 x 11", 298 pages, $35

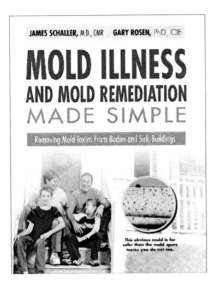

Book • $26.50

Mold Illness and Mold Remediation Made Simple: Removing Mold Toxins from Bodies and Sick Buildings

By James Schaller, M.D. and Gary Rosen, Ph.D.

Indoor mold toxins are much more dangerous and prevalent than most people realize. Visible mold in and around your house is far less dangerous than the mold you cannot see. Indoor mold toxicity, in addition to causing its own unique set of health problems and symptoms, also greatly contributes to the severity of most chronic illnesses.

In this book, a top physician and experienced contractor team up to help you quickly recover from indoor mold exposure. This book is easy to read with many color photographs and illustrations.

Dr. Schaller is a practicing physician in Florida who has written more than 15 books. He is one of the few physicians in the United States successfully treating mold toxin illness in children and adults.

Dr. Rosen is a biochemist with training under a Nobel Prize winning researcher at UCLA. He has written several books and is an expert in the mold remediation of homes. Dr. Rosen and his family are sensitive to mold toxins so he writes not only from professional experience, but also from personal experience.

Together, the two authors have certification in mold testing, mold remediation, and indoor environmental health. This book is one of the most complete on the subject, and includes discussion of the following topics:

- Potential mold problems encountered in new homes, schools, and jobs.
- Diagnosing mold illness.
- Mold as it relates to dryness and humidity.
- Mold toxins and cancer treatment.
- Mold toxins and relationships.
- Crawlspaces, basements, attics, home cleaning techniques, and vacuums.
- Training your eyes to discern indoor mold.
- Leptin and obesity.
- Appropriate/inappropriate air filters and cleaners.
- How to handle old, musty products, materials and books, and how to safely sterilize them.
- A description of various types of molds, images of them, and their relative toxicity.
- Blood testing and how to use it to find hidden health problems.
- The book is written in a friendly, casual tone that allows easy comprehension and information retention.

"A concise, practical guide on dealing with mold toxins and their effects."

- Bryan Rosner

Many people are affected by mold toxins. Are you? If you can find a smarter or clearer book on this subject, buy it!

Paperback book, 8.5 x 11", 140 pages, $26.50

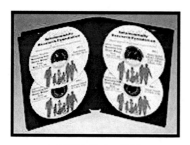

4-DVD Set • $45

Marshall Protocol 4-DVD Set

Recent Chicago Conference:
"Recovering from Chronic Disease"
Recent Hartford Conference:
"30th Anniversary of Lyme"

The Marshall Protocol is not just important, but critical in Lyme Disease recovery. It addresses a part of the Lyme Disease complex that no other treatment, protocol, diet, or supplement can even come close to touching: infection with cell-wall-deficient bacteria.

Borrelia Burgdorferi, the causative bacteria in Lyme Disease, comes in three forms: spirochete, cyst, and cell-wall-deficient. All forms must be addressed to achieve a complete recovery. Spirochetes are successfully killed by rife technology. Cysts can be killed by certain antibiotics (including 5-nitromidizoles and hydroxychloroquine). Cysts can also be exposed and killed by rife therapy with proper treatment timing and planning. However, until the Marshall Protocol, there was not an effective treatment for cell-wall-deficient bacteria.

Conventionally, doctors have tried to use certain types of antibiotics to kill cell-wall-deficient bacteria. Top choices include protein synthesis inhibitors such as the macrolides (Zithromax and Biaxin), the ketolides (Ketek), and the tetracyclines (tetracycline, doxycycline,

> "The Marshall Protocol – especially when combined with rife therapy – fills an important gap in existing Lyme treatment."
> **- Bryan Rosner**

and minocycline). Unfortunately, these antibiotics have been ineffective at worst and only moderately effective at best. According to new research and user reports, the Marshall Protocol successfully targets and kills these cell-wall-deficient bacteria.

This 4-DVD set is exclusively offered by lymebook.com. It was assembled for lymebook.com by the founder of the Autoimmunity Research Foundation, Trevor Marshall, PhD, who also invented the protocol. The DVD set includes video recordings from two conferences of particular interest to Lyme sufferers:

- **DVD 1:** 30th Anniversary of Lyme – Hartford, Connecticut
- **DVD 2-4:** Recovering from Chronic Disease – Chicago, Illinois

James P   Leonard   Lida H   Janet
Kiley, PhD   Jason, PhD   Mattman, PhD   Whitley, PhD

Conference Speakers

Andrew   Trevor G   Meg
Wright, MD   Marshall, PhD   Mangin, RN

4-DVD Set

12+ hours of viewing

Coverage of two Conferences

$45

Researching the Marshall Protocol is an Essential Part of Your Lyme Disease Education!

Physicians Desk Reference (PDR) Books

Most people have heard of *Physicians Desk Reference* (PDR) because, for over 60 years, physicians and researchers have turned to PDR for the latest word on prescription drugs. Today, PDR is considered the standard prescription drug reference and can be found in virtually every physician's office, hospital, and pharmacy in the United States. In fact, nine out of 10 doctors consider PDR their most important drug information reference source. The current edition is over 3,500 pages long (with a full color directory) and weighs more than 5 lbs. It includes comprehensive and up-to-date information on more than 4,000 FDA-approved drugs.

You may not know that Thomson Healthcare, publisher of PDR, offers PDR reference books not only for drugs, but also for herbal and nutritional supplements. No other available books come even 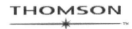 close to the amount of information provided in these PDRs—*PDR for Herbal Medicines* weighs 5 lbs and has over 900 pages, and *PDR for Nutritional Supplements* weighs over 3 lbs and has more than 500 pages.

Lymebook.com carries all three PDRs: *PDR for Prescription Drugs*, *PDR for Herbal Medicines*, and *PDR for Nutritional Supplements.* Although PDR books are typically used by healthcare practitioners, we feel that these resources are also essential for people interested in or recovering from chronic disease. Ownership of PDR books allows you to have at your fingertips information that has historically not been available to the public. Health decisions are always made based on information, and we want you to have the most complete information available.

Would you like to be able to look up all the details of the treatments you are using (or planning to use)? PDR reference books offer the following data on thousands of herbs, supplements and drugs:

- Description and method of action
- Pharmacology
- Available trade names / brands
- Indications and usage
- Research summaries, with recent scientific studies and clinical results
- Contraindications, precautions, adverse reactions

- How supplied
- Scientific literature overviews
- Dosage and administration
- History of use
- Biochemistry and metabolism
- Pharmacokinetics
- Cross references to other helpful data relating to the drug or herb discussed

The PDRs organize the supplements, herbs, and medicines in numerous ways, so you can quickly and easily find the information you need. Multiple color-coded, photo-supported indexes are provided. Supplements and drugs are categorized according to type, name, and health condition, among other differentiators.

"I relied heavily on the PDRs during the research phase of writing my books. Without these books, I'm not sure I could have pulled together the information I needed."

- Bryan Rosner

In addition to information about individual herbs, supplements, and drugs, the PDRs also provide high-level comprehensive health resources such as breakthroughs in the treatment of specific health conditions, anti-aging science, cancer studies, sports medicine, nutrition, and much more.

If you are a doctor, nurse, holistic healthcare provider, or simply a patient wishing to do your own research, these books are must-have resources. They pay for themselves many times over after years of use as reliable reference guides.

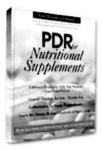

PDR for Nutritional Supplements

This PDR focuses on the following types of supplements:

- Vitamins
- Minerals
- Amino acids
- Hormones
- Lipids
- Glyconutrients
- Probiotics
- Proteins
- Many more!

"In a part of the health field not known for its devotion to rigorous science, [this book] brings to the practitioner and the curious patient a wealth of hard facts."

- Roger Guillemin, M.D., Ph.D., Nobel Laureate in Physiology and Medicine

Book • $69.50

The book also suggests supplements that can help reduce prescription drug side effects, has full-color photographs of various popular commercial formulations (and contact information for the associated suppliers), and so much more! Become educated instead of guessing which supplements to take.

Hardcover book, 11 x 9.3", 575 pages, $69.50

PDR for Herbal Medicines

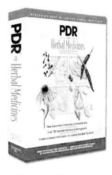

PDR for Herbal Medicines is very well organized and presents information on hundreds of common and uncommon herbs and herbal preparations. Indications and usage are examined with regard to homeopathy, Indian and Chinese medicine, and unproven (yet popular) applications.

In an area of healthcare so unstudied and vulnerable to hearsay and hype, this scientifically referenced book allows you to find out the real story behind the herbs lining the walls of your local health food store.

Use this reference before spending money on herbal products!

Book • $69.50

Hardcover book, 11 x 9.3", 988 pages, $69.50

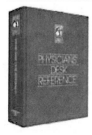

PDR for Prescription Drugs

With more than 3,000 pages, this is the most comprehensive and respected book in the world on over 4,000 drugs. Drugs are indexed by both brand and generic name (in the same convenient index) and also by manufacturer and product category. This PDR provides usage information and warnings, drug interactions, plus a detailed, full-color directory with descriptions and cross references for the drugs. A new format allows dramatically improved readability and easier access to the information you need now.

Book • $99.50

Hardcover book, 12.5 x 9.5", 3533 pages, $99.50

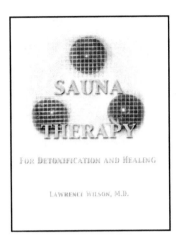

Book • $19.95

Sauna Therapy for Detoxification and Healing

By Lawrence Wilson, MD

This book is the single most authoritative source on sauna therapy. It includes construction plans for a low-cost electric light sauna. The book is well referenced with an extensive bibliography.

Sauna therapy, especially with an electric light sauna, is one of the most powerful, safe and cost-effective methods of natural healing. It is especially important today due to extensive exposure to toxic metals and chemicals.

Fifteen chapters cover sauna benefits, physiological effects, protocols, cautions, healing reactions, and many other aspects of sauna therapy.

Dr. Wilson is an instructor of Biochemistry, Hair Mineral Analysis, Sauna Therapy and Jurisprudence at various colleges and universities including Yamuni Institute of the Healing Arts (Maurice, LA), University of Natural Medicine (Santa Fe, NM), Natural Healers Academy (Morristown, NJ), and Westbrook University (West Virginia). His books are used as textbooks at East-West School of Herbology and Ohio College of Natural Health.

Paperback book, 8.5 x 11", 167 pages, $19.95

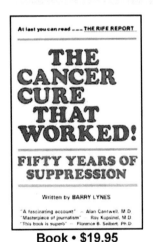

Book • $19.95

Over 50,000 Copies Sold!

The Cancer Cure That Worked: Fifty Years of Suppression

At Last You Can Read... The Rife Report

By Barry Lynes

Investigative journalism at its best. Barry Lynes takes readers on an exciting journey into the life work of Royal Rife. **In 2008, we became the official distributor for this book. Call or visit us online for wholesale terms.**

"A fascinating account..."
-Alan Cantwell, MD

"This book is superb."
-Florence B. Seibert, PhD

"Barry Lynes is one of the greatest health reporters in our country. With the assistance of John Crane, longtime friend and associate of Roy Rife, Barry has produced a masterpiece..." -Roy Kupsinel, M.D., editor of *Health Consciousness Journal*

Paperback book, 5 x 8", 169 pages, $19.95

Rife Video Documentary
2-Part DVD Set, Produced by
Zero Zero Two Productions

Must-Have DVD set for your Rife technology education!

In 1999, a stack of forgotten audio tapes was discovered. On the tapes were the voices of several people at the center of the events which are the subject of this documentary: a revolutionary treatment for cancer and a practical cure for all infectious disease.

The audio tapes were over 40 years old. The voices on them had almost faded, nearly losing key details of perhaps the most important medical story of the 20th Century.

But due to the efforts of the Kinnaman Foundation, the faded tapes have been restored and the voices on them recovered. So now, even though the participants have all passed away...

...they can finally tell their story.

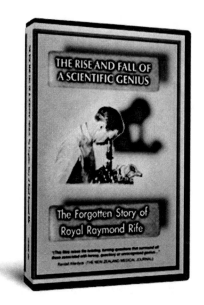

2-part DVD Set • $39.95

"These videos are great. We show them at the Annual Rife International Health Conference."
-Richard Loyd, Ph.D.

"A mind-shifting experience for those of us indoctrinated with a conventional view of biology."
-Townsend Letter for Doctors and Patients

In the summer of 1934 at a special medical clinic in La Jolla, California, sixteen patients withering from terminal disease were given a new lease on life. It was the first controlled application of a new electronic treatment for cancer: the Beam Ray Machine.

Within ninety days all sixteen patients walked away from the clinic, signed-off by the attending doctors as cured.

What followed the incredible success of this revolutionary treatment was not a welcoming by the scientific community, but a sad tale of its ultimate suppression.

The Rise and Fall of a Scientific Genius documents the scientific ignorance, official corruption, and personal greed directed at the inventor of the Beam Ray Machine, Royal Raymond Rife, forcing him and his inventions out of the spotlight and into obscurity. **Just converted from VHS to DVD and completely updated.**

Do not miss this opportunity to educate yourself about the history of rife technology!

Includes bonus DVD with interviews and historical photographs! Produced in Canada.

2 DVD-set, including bonus DVD, $39.95

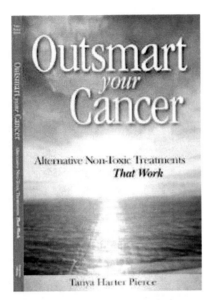

Book and Audio CD • $24.50

Outsmart Your Cancer: Alternative Non-Toxic Treatments That Work

By Tanya Harter Pierce

Note: Although Lymebook.com primarily focuses on books and resources for Lyme Disease, we know that cancer affects many of our customers. Consequently, we offer this excellent book/audio CD set on alternative cancer therapy.

Publisher's Remarks:

Why BLUDGEON cancer to death with common conventional treatments that can be toxic and harmful to your entire body?

When you OUTSMART your cancer, only the cancer cells die — NOT your healthy cells!

OUTSMART YOUR CANCER: Alternative Non-Toxic Treatments That Work is an easy guide to successful non-toxic treatments for cancer that you can obtain right now! In it, you will read real-life stories of people who have completely recovered from their advanced or late-stage lung cancer, breast cancer, prostate cancer, kidney cancer, brain cancer, childhood leukemia, and other types of cancer using effective non-toxic approaches.

This book explains the successful approaches these people used. It also gives you the resources to obtain these treatments right now, including a list of phone numbers and answers to questions about financial cost.

You will also learn other valuable information, such as:

> "As a doctor practicing alternative medicine, I recommend this book to anyone that is involved with cancer."
> - Dr. L. Durrett

- The unique characteristics of cancer cells that can be exploited to "outsmart" cancer.
- How to evaluate mainstream conventional treatments and what questions to ask your doctor.
- What women need to know about their hormones and cancer.
- How to alkalize your body and why this matters, both for prevention and treatment of cancer.
- Many of the causes of cancer that are increasingly common in our modern world.
- How and why many of the best alternative treatments for cancer have been suppressed.
- How to cope with the fear that comes with a cancer diagnosis.

Plus, *OUTSMART YOUR CANCER* is one of the few books in print today that gives a complete description of the amazing formula called "Protocel," which has produced incredible cancer recoveries over the past 20 years! A supporting audio CD is included with this book. Pricing = $19.95 book + $5.00 CD.

Paperback book, 6 x 9", 437 pages, with audio CD, $24.95

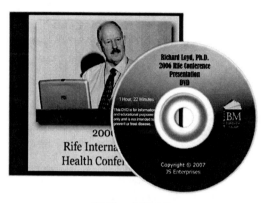

Richard Loyd, Ph.D., presents at the Rife International Health Conference in Seattle

Watch this DVD to gain a better understanding of the technical details of rife technology.

DVD • $19.95

Dr. Loyd, who earned a Ph.D. in nutrition, has researched and experimented with numerous electrotherapeutic devices, including the Rife/Bare unit, various EMEM machines, F-Scan, BioRay, magnetic pulsers, Doug Machine, and more. Dr. Loyd also has a wealth of knowledge in the use of herbs and supplements to support Rife electromagnetics.

By watching this DVD, you will discover the nuts and bolts of some very important, yet little known, principles of rife machine operation, including:

- Gating, sweeping, session time
- Square vs. sine wave
- DC vs. AC frequencies
- Duty cycle
- Octaves and scalar octaves

- Voltage variations and radio frequencies
- Explanation of the spark gap
- Contact vs. radiant mode
- Stainless vs. copper contacts
- A unique look at various frequency devices

DVD, 59 minutes, $19.95

The 2008 Lyme Disease Annual Report, by Bryan Rosner and Contributing Writers

This book serves as Bryan Rosner's annual newsletter.

The 2008 report covers numerous topics, including glyconutrient supplementation, updates on rife machine treatment planning and machine manufacturers, evidence supporting the existence of chronic Lyme Disease as a real medical condition, statistics indicating the presence of Lyme Disease on all continents of the planet, and much more. Includes articles by 6 contributing writers: **James Schaller, M.D., Richard Brand, M.D., Sue Vogan, Ginger Savely, FNP-C, Tami Duncan, Susan Williams, and Richard Loyd, Ph.D.** Stay up to date!

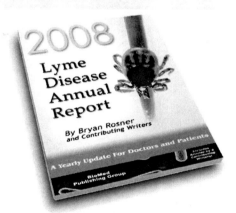

Paperback Book • $19.95

Paperback book, 7 x 10", 168 pages, $19.95

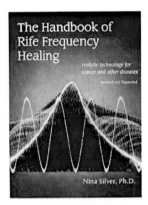

Book • $60

The Handbook of Rife Frequency Healing: Holistic Technology for Cancer and Other Diseases

By Nenah Sylver, PhD

This is the most complete, authoritative Rife technology handbook in the world. Weighing over 2 lbs., and 448 pages long, a broad range of topics are covered:

- Little-known differences between allopathic (Western) medicine and holistic health care
- Royal Raymond Rife's life, inventions, ideas and relationships
- Frequently Asked Questions about Rife sessions and equipment, with extensive session information
- Ground-breaking information on strengthening and supporting the body, based on years of research by the author
- A 200-page, cross-referenced Frequency Directory including hundreds of health conditions
- Bibliography, Three Appendices, Historical Photos, and MUCH MORE!

Paperback book, 8.5 x 11", 430 pages, $60

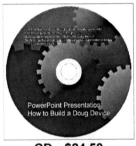

CD • $24.50

PowerPoint Presentation on CD
How to Build a Coil Machine

Of all rife machines used to fight Lyme Disease, the Coil Machine (also known as the Doug Device or QSC1850HD Device) has the longest and most established track record. This PowerPoint presentation was put together by the husband of a Lyme Disease sufferer who built the machine for his wife. It provides construction information, parts sourcing, and a detailed schematic. Now you can build your own Coil Machine!

Microsoft PowerPoint Presentation on CD, $24.50

CPSIA information can be obtained at www.ICGtesting.com
Printed in the USA
LVOW131441240911

247674LV00003B/3/P